Adventures in Obstetrics

Helping women deliver their babies with other humorous and heartfelt stories

Gary Matsumura MD

Simon & Deschanel

Fairfield, California

Simon & Deschanel

Fairfield, California

garymatsumura.com

The following stories are based on my personal and professional experiences as a physician. However, to protect the privacy and confidentiality of my patients, I have changed or omitted details, such as names, dates, locations, and medical conditions. In some cases, I have also combined multiple patient experiences into one composite story, while staying true to the essence of each individual's experience.

Project management and interior layout by Wonderlady Books

Adventures in Obstetrics: Helping Women Deliver Their Babies with Other Humorous and Heartfelt Stories / Gary Matsumura, MD. — 1st ed.

ISBN 979-8-9903323-0-0 paperback

ISBN 979-8-9903323-1-7 ebook

Library of Congress Control Number: 2024905766

Dedication

This book is dedicated to Kathy. You are the unwavering light that helped me find my way when I would stumble.

Acknowledgements

I would like to thank the following individuals for their editing expertise: Kelley Sewell, Mark Obmascik, Monica Wesolowska, and Ross Plotkin.

I also want to acknowledge Ruth Schwartz for her publishing expertise, as well as her eagle eye final edits.

Table of Contents

Introduction

In high school, I wanted to be a rock star. What seventeen-year-old kid in the seventies didn't? It wasn't something one would necessarily say out loud. It could lead to encouragement at best and derisive comments at worst. It would be like saying you wanted to be a movie star. Well, who wouldn't?

I found myself in Riverside, California, registering as a freshman at La Sierra University in the fall of 1970. As I waited my turn, I eavesdropped on the young woman ahead of me, talking to a counselor. She was an English major, and she could not get into an English class that she wanted due to a scheduling conflict. In total frustration, she said, "This is not going to work out! Let's change my major to pre-med."

When it was my turn, the counselor told me his name was Dr. Botimer and that he was a chemistry teacher. He was a slim, handsome fellow with graying hair. He asked me if I had chosen a major. I said, "Yes, it is music, but before we get into that, what about that previous student changing her major from English to pre-med so capriciously?" We looked to be sure she was out of earshot, and then we both laughed. I then winked and said, "Kids today, what ya gonna do?" Three months later, I changed my major to pre-med.

I chose to become a doctor because I wanted to be respected and not have to worry about money. As a young man, I remember reading that being a doctor earned more respect than any other profession other than being a Supreme Court justice.

We respect doctors—we have to. We all have to see one at some point. They literally hold our lives in their hands, starting in the delivery room. Today people have a fear of gluten and vaccines but not so much of anesthesia. We wouldn't be able to be put to sleep for surgery if we didn't feel confident that we would be waking up again.

Patients think that physicians have everything under control. Doctors ooze confidence. Their rigorous training, expertise, and dedication almost guarantee a favorable outcome, or so we believe.

Doctors are calm, cautious, and don't show panic. Whenever I call for an emergency cesarean section, I know that all hell is about to break loose. I don't want to make the patient anxious, so I whisper in the patient's ear: "Your baby will be coming out of you in just a few minutes as I am about to call for an emergency cesarean section. When I do, it is going to look like a Chinese fire drill around here. I am allowed to use that racial slur because I am Asian." I smile, and the patient smiles. I then call for the emergency cesarean, and all hell breaks loose.

What you don't know is that there are times when doctors are more anxious than the patient.

I recall having a patient in labor with a prolapsed umbilical cord. That is when the cord starts delivering out of the vagina before the baby's head, and then the cord gets trapped between the fetal head and the mother's pelvis, cutting off the blood supply to the baby. The fetal heart rate was already dangerously low when the nurse noted the slowly pulsating cord was presenting in the vagina. The baby needs to deliver in the next few minutes before she suffers from a lack of oxygen, but it may take longer than that to get to the operating room from the labor room. Even then, the patient needs anesthesia before the cesarean can start. As we transport the patient from the labor room to the operating room, I go through some of the steps of the cesarean in my mind. I think, "Once I have the scalpel in my hand, and the patient is anesthetized, I can probably get this baby out in one minute. Entering the uterus that quickly with the scalpel, I need to be careful not to cut the baby accidentally."

I tell the patient, "Keep your hands and feet close to your body so that they won't get pinched when we go through the doors. I know it looks like we are in a panic, but we do this all the time." The patient tries to put on a brave face. Her voice is shaking, but she manages to say, "I'm fine, doctor. I trust you."

There are unwieldy poles on wheels holding infusion pumps (pumps that allow different fluids and medications into the patient through plastic tubing). The patient's bed gets stuck in the doorway with the infusion pumps. The problem is trying to get too many things out through the door at once. An infusion pump alarm goes off. I am panicked inside, but I calmly say, "Turn off that pump and disconnect it. Pull the pump back into the room and let the bed go first."

This book will show you that we physicians appear self-confident but are often in doubt. We do our best, and almost all of our patients have a good outcome. Some do not.

I have always brought humor into my practice of obstetrics. Humor helps relax the patient, the staff, and me as well. It immediately lets the patient see that I am just as human as she is. I will try to safely guide her baby out of her uterus and into her arms. At that moment, humor helps break the tension. This book will introduce you to the joys and heartbreak of caring for women. In childbirth, there is a time to laugh and to cry.

Chapter 1

Suzanne, the Plans They Made

My patient was in labor. Her vaginal bleeding was becoming excessive, so I had to address the issue before she became alarmed.

"Please lift your bottom so I can change the pad underneath you. Lift up, up," I said to my laboring patient Jacquie as I quickly removed one pad and replaced it with a clean one. Jacquie's husband, Mike, seeing the purple-stained pad with large clots on it, said, "Yuck, nobody wants to see that."

"I'm sorry, but we are going to have to do a cesarean," I continued. "I'm sure you've noticed that your bleeding is a bit heavy, and the trickling of blood shows no sign of letting up."

Jacquie replied, "Well, that's okay. I never really wanted to deliver vaginally. I didn't make a big deal about it before because everyone encouraged me to deliver vaginally throughout my pregnancy. I'm relieved."

In her first pregnancy, Jacquie had a breech presentation of her baby. Breech presentation means her baby was lined up to come out buttocks first instead of head first, which is the normal presentation.

During that pregnancy, Jacquie had made an appointment at the hospital for an attempt at turning the baby to the head-down position. Mike and I gathered around Jacquie as she reclined in her hospital bed. I used the ultrasound to confirm that the baby was still breech, which it was. I then told Mike not to freak out as I was about to put my hands on Jacquie's tummy and would try to rotate the baby's body 180 degrees. As I successfully moved the baby's head from the top of Jacquie's abdomen to the bottom, Mike's eyes got very large. I joked to him, "Don't try this at home." The attempt to turn the baby was over in about a minute.

Unfortunately, when Jacquie went into labor, her baby's heart rate dropped to a dangerous level and she ended up having a cesarean anyway.

In this pregnancy, the baby was not breech, so I encouraged Jacquie to try a vaginal delivery. If she were to deliver vaginally, she would avoid major surgery.

In one of her prenatal visits, she had reluctantly gone along with the plan to deliver vaginally. However, she had told me, "The advantage of having a scheduled cesarean is that one does not have to deal with the uncertainty of not knowing what day labor will start or how I will deal with the pain. My sister was sent home from the hospital three times. Each time the doctor told her that although she was having contractions, she was not yet in labor."

In a later prenatal visit, she said, "I am concerned that I will labor for days and then still end up with a cesarean."

"That is always a possibility," I replied, "but what if you only labor for one day and are ready to go home the following day?" Jacquie had smiled but looked skeptical. She had shaken her head as if to say, "I'm not buying it."

There is a large pad that we place under patients' buttocks as they lie in their labor beds. It looks more like a painter's small drop cloth than a pad. They are usually blue, and we call them Chux. They are absorbent on the patient side and waterproof on the other. They are handy in absorbing amniotic fluid, blood, and anything else that may come out of the vagina, rectum, or bladder. I asked Jacquie's nurse to monitor the chux by weighing them to estimate how much blood loss there was.

Due to excess bleeding, the Chux had been changed every twenty minutes. Even Jacquie and Mike could see that she would eventually run out of blood if the bleeding continued.

It was my job to address the problem before the couple became alarmed. I had been walking into their labor room frequently so that the couple could see that I was attentive to the issue. Speaking calmly, I reassured them that this was a routine problem that I could easily manage. In most cases, that was true. Jacquie had only been in labor for a few hours.

My anxiety level had increased with the bleeding, but Jacquie's had decreased with the decision to have a cesarean. She wanted to deliver and put this anxious time of waiting behind her. She just wanted to hold her baby in her arms.

I then whispered to Nurse Lee, "Go ahead and tell the staff to prepare for an emergency cesarean." I then told Jacquie, "The staff will now look like they are in a panic preparing for your delivery, but I can assure you that this is routine. They do this all the time. I have done thousands of cesareans. We will now take you to a different room where we do cesareans. I will be with you the entire time to give you reassurance. I will distract you with amusing stories, jokes, and I may even sing to you." Jacquie had a look of concern, but she squeezed my hand and said, "I trust you."

In the operating room, I told Jacquie, "Please help us help you slide onto the operating table." I immediately regretted using the word "operating." Jacquie slid onto the table but then started screaming, "I can't do this! I can't do this! Stop everything! I need Valium!"

I told Jacquie, "I would rather not give you Valium at this point, as it will go right to the baby, and it will be on board when the baby tries to take her first breath."

I asked the anesthesiologist to give Jacquie some Phenergan. Jacquie asked, "Is that like a cousin to Valium?"

I said, "Think of it as Valium's cousin's roommate. I could see that the anesthesiologist Richard was smiling even though his mask was on.

The anesthesiologist then said in a loud voice, "The Phenergan is in."

I asked Jacquie if she was feeling any better. She said, "Yes, actually, thank you."

I thought to myself, "Never underestimate the value of a placebo." I have experienced the boost from drinking a cup of coffee only to find out later that it was decaf.

Jacquie's face was now behind a blue paper drape, so I could not see her, but I could still talk to her. "I used to tell inappropriate stories in the O.R.", I said to Jacquie, "but I quit after taking a class on harassment. Since I stopped telling those stories, my surgical assistant says that I have become so boring, she is thinking about retiring early." I added, "Nevertheless, in your honor, I will tell one last inappropriate joke to distract you." Although the nurses had masks on, I could see their eyes rolling.

I started, "My wife asked me if I was having sex behind her back." I said, 'Well, who did you think that was?'"

The room went quiet except for a few muffled chuckles. The staff did not want to get into trouble for participating in an inappropriate joke. What if someone were to take offense, and I ended up getting reported? Richard, the anesthesiologist, was originally from China. He would often not understand the subtlety of an American joke. At that point, he said, "I don't get it."

Jacquie burst out laughing, causing everyone in the O.R. to laugh. Jacquie appeared for the moment to be relaxed enough for us to proceed with the surgery.

At that point, I was careful not to say to the surgical tech, "Scalpel, please." If Jacquie heard that, she might have freaked out again. I instead glanced at the nurse and said, "Bard-Parker, please." That is a brand of scalpel.

I am always circumspect with my informal banter during a cesarean as the patient is awake and attended to by her partner. They are carefully listening to everything said in the O.R. as they await the first cry of their newborn. If I make a small error, such as cutting into a blood vessel during the surgery, I never say, "Oops." Instead, I say, "There," or "Okay."

Assisting me with the surgery that night was surgical Registered Nurse First Assistant (RNFA) Suzanne. I liked working with Suzanne because she would politely laugh at all of my jokes.

Suzanne's last name is Gourioux. We had another nurse who worked with us from France. She was fluent in the French language. One day she told Suzanne that she was not pronouncing her last name correctly. When the French nurse pronounced Suzanne's name, she made sounds that an English-speaking person would never produce. It sounded as though she was trying to say, Goodyear while eating a mouthful of soft cheese. None of us could pronounce the name correctly, including Suzanne. We finally gave up. My last name is Matsumura. I imagine if I tried to pronounce my surname in Japan, there would be some raised eyebrows.

Whenever I see Suzanne, I always sing her a line from a James Taylor song. I sing, *Suzanne, the plans they made put an end to you.* Those of us listening to the radio in the 1970s can remember what was going on in our lives when that song was popular. Suzanne always found it to be a bit amusing that I would sing that one line to her. I never gave any explanation as to the origin of that line.

Suzanne related the following story to me as she assisted in the cesarean. "I was talking to my mother on the phone yesterday, and I told her, 'There is this obstetrician who works with me. Every time he sees me, or even talks to me on the phone, I remind him of a song, and he sings, *Suzanne, the plans they made put an end to you.* My mother then said, 'I named you after that song.'"

After hearing that, I felt very nostalgic and quietly, under my mask, sang:

"*Just yesterday morning, they let me know you were gone. Suzanne, the plans they made put an end to you. I walked out this morning, and I wrote down this song....*"

At that point, those in the room familiar with the song started singing along. Even the surgical tech, who is younger than my children, sang along as she passed instruments.

It was very quiet after the singing. I broke the silence with, "Jacquie, are you okay with us singing at your delivery?"

She replied, "I was quite anxious when the surgery started, but then I got caught up in your story. I then thought, 'well, things must be going pretty smoothly if they can sing during my surgery.'"

I laughed, "Well, you'd be surprised. I also sing when the surgery is not going well."

I pulled a baby girl out of Jacquie's uterus. The baby had a lusty cry, which is always a relief to the parents. It is not just the parents that welcome the newborn's first cry. The entire operating room gives an inaudible sigh of relief at that point—the whole atmosphere of the room changes. The rest of the cesarean is much more relaxed. At that point, we just put things back the way they were. Jacquie's anxiety appeared to be gone entirely, even though the surgery was not over. Mike held their squinting newborn as Jacquie said to her baby girl, "How are you? We've been waiting for you." I started sewing the uterus closed.

Since the stressful part of the case was over, I engaged my assistant in casual conversation. I asked Suzanne if she could name the four Beatles. Suzanne is much younger than me but well into her thirties. My guess was that she could list them all.

Suzanne asked, "Is one of them James Taylor?" The room went dead quiet. I stopped operating. I carefully put my suture down on the surgical stand that holds the instruments. The surgical tech looked at me as if to say, "Why have you stopped operating?" I did not believe what I had just heard. I felt as though I was about to wake up from a dream. The patient's voice from behind the drapes broke the silence, "Are you f**king kidding me?" Suddenly everyone in the room started laughing. I asked our anesthesiologist if he could name the four Beatles. He named them all, ending with Paul McCarthy. I said, "Close enough."

At Jacquie's postpartum visit six weeks later, she told me that she had not been familiar with James Taylor but that the song now meant a lot to her and Mike as I had introduced them to it at the most memorable moment of their lives. They purchased the music and planned to play the song for their daughter in the future.

I remember in 1970 thinking that the lyrics were quite sad. I later learned that the Suzanne mentioned in the song was James Taylor's friend and had committed suicide. Carole King had played piano for the recording. A line in the song goes: *"I've seen lonely times when I could not find a friend...."* That sad thought moved Carole King. She could not imagine not being able to find a single friend. She decided to write a song in response. She named her song, "You've Got a Friend."

The song "Fire and Rain" is about James Taylor attempting to make sense of the world as a young man. It meant a lot to me as a struggling pre-med student in Southern California in the 1970s. I was discouraged, as I had received rejection letters from all the medical schools I had applied to and did not have a backup plan. The song spoke to me and my generation.

Chapter 2

Oh My God, Your English Is So Good

I first noticed that foreigners thought I was from Japan many years ago when I took my family to Paris. I had rented an apartment near the Eiffel Tower. I would wake each morning, admire the most recognizable monument in Europe, and then head for the boulangerie near our apartment to bring back pastries for my family's breakfast.

This bakery had beautiful pastries in the display window. One could not help but stop and admire the beautiful fresh framboise and citron tarts even if you weren't going to make a purchase. It was like walking by kittens in a store window. Each morning I would greet the baker with, "Bonjour, Monsieur Duquesne. Comment allez-vous?" He would then respond with something I could not understand. I would then ask him to repeat himself, but more slowly: "Excusez-moi, repetez s'il vous plait, lentement." I would still not understand his response, so I would just say okay in French: "D'accord." He was impressed that I knew the word "D'accord," and he would laugh.

I had been warned that the French might be rude to American tourists, but I found this baker to be very friendly. I assumed that most Americans do not make an effort to try to speak French.

This trip to Paris was many years ago when it was common to use traveler's checks. One morning I noticed I was running low on cash, so I asked the baker if he would cash a traveler's check for me. "Acceptez-vous des cheques de voyage?" I asked.

He asked me the denomination of the check I was trying to cash. I told him it was for $100. He said the amount was too large and that he would not cash it.

I then said, "Well, you French are rather arrogant considering we saved your ass in World War II." He understood my English, got a shocked look on his face, and said, "Oh mon Dieu, I thought you were Japonaise."

I replied indignantly, "No, je suis Americain!" I started to laugh, and he could see that I had been kidding him. Fortunately, he had a sense of humor. I would not have wanted to start an international incident. He cashed my check.

I am Japanese, but not really. Although I am of Japanese ancestry, I am no more Japanese than my wife is Hungarian. My wife always thought she was Polish as her mother's maiden name was Kibosh. More recently, however, we found out that my wife's ancestors were Hungarian. Now that my wife knows that she is Hungarian, it has not made a big difference in her life. We have a three-foot globe in our home. I could see that my wife was having difficulty finding Hungary on it. I told her to find Romania and turn left. Knowing that she is Hungarian has not made her more interested in Hungary than before she had this information. She cannot speak a single word of Hungarian unless you count goulash.

Other than English, the only other language I can speak is Spanish. Since I was a practicing OB/GYN physician in California, I learned to speak some Spanish out of necessity. My Hispanic patients were often surprised that a "japones" could talk to them in their native tongue. My Spanish is very basic, but I could immediately see the gratitude in my patient's smile. We had a telephone translator service available to us, but the patient felt much more welcome if the doctor made an effort to learn her language.

When it comes to Japanese, I can barely speak enough to order in a Japanese restaurant. The first time I entered a sushi restaurant, the sushi chef startled me with a loud greeting of "Irasshaimase!" I responded with an equally loud, "What did you just say?" I think that irasshaimase means, "Welcome to the store!" or "Come on in!"

I have had many native Japanese women come to see me as patients. Their faces immediately drop with disappointment when they realize that I don't speak Japanese. Somehow the expectation is that if I have a Japanese surname, I should be fluent in Japanese.

I have often asked myself why people would expect me to speak Japanese. When one meets an African American, one does not ever ask if he can still speak his original African language. One would not expect an American named Murphy to speak any Gaelic. Well, to be fair, I don't think the Murphys in Ireland speak Gaelic anymore.

I think the difference is that we came from the old country later than African and European Americans. Also, our physical features set us apart. Sometimes a Jew could pass for a German, but an Asian could not.

I have lived in Fairfield, California, for most of my life. It is one of the most diverse counties in the United States. We have no majority race. Mostly, we are Caucasians, Hispanics, Asians, and Blacks. My tennis instructor was waiting to pick up his daughter at Rodriguez High School one day. He noted that the students leaving school at the end of the day were of such mixed race that an observer would not be able to determine their ethnic backgrounds. He also noted that no one cared. This is one of the things about Fairfield that appeals to him.

I imagine that the U.S. and the world will eventually look like our community. Our American society is becoming more liberal as time goes on. In 1958, only 4% of Americans accepted interracial marriage, but by 2013, 87% approved it. Gallup has not bothered to repeat the survey since.

Although I am 100 percent of Japanese ancestry and look the part, it is more challenging to determine what my children are. My daughter has red hair and green eyes. My son has brown hair and brown eyes.

As the races intermarry, we will form a more homogenous-looking society. But that day is not today. When I travel in Europe, people assume that I am from Japan. When I am in Japan, they expect me to be able to speak Japanese. Even in the U.S., I have been mistaken for a Japanese tourist. I can feel as though I am a man without a country, from neither here nor there. Our assumptions about people are often based solely on appearance.

I have asked myself if there are any advantages to having the appearance of being from another country. I imagine one could pretend that one does not speak anything but Japanese in certain situations, but that would not come up very often. It could be advantageous when visiting a country where Americans are not welcome, possibly an Arab country. Maybe I should have entertained the idea of a career with the State Department.

When I visited Japan for the first time, the people there could not always tell that I was an American. There, people would often start speaking to me in Japanese. I assumed this was going to happen, so I committed a phrase to memory, "Nihongo-ga wakari masen." That means, "I don't understand Japanese." The person I spoke to would then get a puzzled look on his face, but I was helpless to explain why I couldn't speak Japanese. My friend Dr. Levine says the Japanese people must think that I am mentally retarded. It is evident to them that I am old enough to be speaking.

I have a physician friend that is a Mormon. He spent several years in Japan as a missionary. He suggested that we both vacation in Japan sometime, and he would go as my translator. What a sight that would be, as he is blond and speaks fluent Japanese.

My wife cannot tell the difference between the various Asian ethnic groups. She cannot tell the difference between a Filipino, Chinese, Japanese, Thai, or Vietnamese. I asked her if there were any races she could readily identify. She said she could recognize blacks. Also, she could point out a Mexican if he was wearing a sombrero.

I can usually tell the difference between the different Asian races. I can even tell the difference between first-generation (Issei) and second-generation (Nisei) Japanese Americans. I am a fourth-generation (Yonsei) Japanese American. If you are at Disneyland and you see four Japanese males walking abreast, all in suits and ties, you can assume that these men are Japanese nationals. Endless bowing is another clue.

A few years ago, I took my family to the incredible ruins of Angkor Wat in Cambodia. Unfortunately, I had not done enough research before embarking on that trip, so we arrived during monsoon season. It was sweltering and humid. I found myself sitting on the steps of a 900-year-old-temple in the midday sun, taking a break and drinking from my bottle of water.

Next to me, also sitting and taking a break, were two young men from the Netherlands. Asian tourists surrounded us. One of the men remarked to the other, "Do you know how many more of them there are than us in the world?" I responded, in perfect English, "There are a billion more of us, and someday we're taking over." They looked at me in astonishment for one uncomfortable moment, as they were not expecting me to understand English. I then said, "Aw, I'm just messing with you." We had a good laugh.

Our hotel was located close to the ancient temples in a lovely town called Siem Reap. We would come back to our hotel around 4 pm each day so that my wife could shop.

My wife finds shopping to be the best part of tourism. Once, we visited Blarney Castle in Ireland. She found a vast gift shop there with many high-quality woolen goods for sale. She decided this would be an excellent opportunity to do her Christmas shopping. Several hours passed. Before she had time to see Blarney Castle, it was time to board the tour bus and head toward our next destination. My wife had no regrets. She said, "In Europe, castles and cathedrals are commonplace, but shopping is always a new adventure."

I don't care for shopping in Cambodia or anywhere else. Silk scarves can only hold my attention for so long. I do enjoy talking to young salesladies. I ask them if they have any souvenirs to sell. Since that is all they sell, they respond with an enthusiastic, "Yes, yes, I make you good price!"

The vendors in Siem Reap will often try to get you to leave a neighboring vendor's stall to buy from them. They call out, "Same, same but better," or "Same, same but different." It is such a common saying that they print those phrases on tee shirts.

In her late teens, I found an attractive woman at the back of a shopping area looking very bored, as most tourists did not venture back to her market area. She had just greeted a Japanese couple in Japanese, but she welcomed me in English. "You want to buy?" she asked. I asked her how she knew I was an American and not a Japanese tourist. She said she could tell I was an American by the way I walked. I said, "Really, do I have a swagger like John Wayne?" She knew who John Wayne was from watching American movies. I decided to do my impersonation of John Wayne for her. I walked back up to her with a wide stance, and in a deep, slow voice, I said, "Konichiwa, pilgrim." She laughed.

My son Eric then came by looking for me. I told the young woman, "This is my son, Eric." She was very playful and said, "Are you sure? He no look like you." I laughed and said, "Yes, I am sure." She then smiled and said, "Are you one hundred percent?" I squeezed her and said, "You are very funny." She then said, "Where your wife?" I said, "She is down there looking for scarves." She responded with, "Oh, oh, she want to buy?"

When it comes to vacationing in the United States, my favorite destination is Ko Olina, Oahu. I could see from my sixth-floor condo that the hot tub spa by the pool was empty. I like using the spa, but I prefer not having to share it with other vacationers. I quickly changed into my swim attire, but by the time I got to the spa, two older Caucasian women were already in the water. (By older, I mean my age.)

The women did not have the jet bubbles on, and I find the bubbles to be the best part of the spa experience. I did not want to be rude and turn on the bubbles. These women apparently preferred to have the bubbles off. Maybe they enjoyed the quiet of having the bubbles off so they could talk.

Every so often, I would splash a bit so they would have to recognize that I was in the spa with them. I was hoping one of them would ask me if I would like the bubbles turned on. Finally, one of the women got out of the spa and went to the control knob. She thought that I did not speak English. She turned to me and asked, "You like, you like?"

I immediately became indignant. How dare she? Did she think that I was "fresh off the boat?" I decided that I would have to teach this woman a lesson. However, if there is one racial stereotype that I believe in, it is that the Japanese are non-confrontational. Although my ancestors arrived here by boat in the nineteenth century, that part of me had come through the generations. I would try to teach this woman a lesson—but in a nice way.

I responded, "Me like, me like." I then added, "Yo quero mucho."

The woman now looked confused. She asked, "Where are you from?"

I couldn't resist showing off my command of the English language. I said, "I come from the land down under, where women glow and men plunder."

I thought she would next say, "Does that mean you are from Australia?"

I was wrong. She then asked, "Isn't that one of the lyrics from the band *Men at Work*?"

I said, "Yes, it is."

She asked, "Whatever happened to them?"

I responded with a serious look on my face, "They are all unemployed."

I don't know why this one time I had become so annoyed. I think it is because these were Americans, and

I am an American. To me, it would be like an Englishman asking Queen Elizabeth II if she was from England.

On arriving in Amsterdam, I decided that my first destination would be the famous *Rijksmuseum*. I found the curator and asked, "Would you please direct me to Rembrandt's *The Night Watch*? Since I was in college, I have admired that painting and never dreamed I would ever actually get to see the genuine article. I would also like to see some Vermeer paintings. I would love to stay and see all that your museum has to offer but after seeing those paintings, I must be off to see the other wonderful sights of your city such as the Van Gogh Museum, Ann Frank's house, and last but not least, the red-light district. I'm sorry for talking so fast, but I am very excited."

She looked at me in astonishment and said, "Oh my God, your English is so good! You have almost no accent! How did you learn to speak English so good?"

I replied, "Did you mean to ask how I learned to speak English so <u>well</u>?"

She anxiously said, "Yes, yes, how did you learn to speak English so well?"

At first, I just stood there. I didn't understand what she was saying to me. Why wouldn't I speak English well? Then I realized that she thought I was a Japanese tourist and assumed I would be speaking Japanese or possibly English with a strong accent.

I laughed and said, "Well, I was listening to an English language disc and fell asleep. When I awoke, I was speaking like this." The curator's mouth dropped.

She then said that she had a few questions for me if I had time for them. I said, "Bien sur," which means, "Of course," in French. She looked at me as if to say, "Whoa, don't tell me you speak French too."

She asked me what I liked about Amsterdam. I told her that there was so much to see and yet it was a much more relaxed city than, say Paris. Paris is exciting, but exhausting. I also told her I enjoyed being in a city that tolerates drugs and prostitution, and accepted homosexuals before it became fashionable to do so.

She then thanked me. Maybe at that point, I should have mentioned that I couldn't speak Japanese.

Later that same evening, my family and I had dinner in a Malaysian restaurant. After dinner, the sun was still reasonably high in the sky, so we decided to walk to the red-light district. Although it was a red-light district, it didn't seem that seedy. It appeared to be a clean and safe area with many tourists walking around. Like much of Amsterdam, it was lined with canals.

The old part of Amsterdam city is so very quaint, with its narrow, cobbled streets and 16th-century buildings. As we rounded a corner, there was a church. It shared the road with the prostitutes' windowed storefronts. I could not take my eyes off the church, but it was closed, so I walked around it. My daughter Kristen caught up with me and asked why I was looking at a church instead of the pretty women in the windows.

I said to her, "Kristen, this is the Oude Kerk, or Old Church. I read about this in a guidebook. This stone church was built in the 1300s, and Rembrandt used to attend services here. Look, it has flying buttresses like

Notre Dame in Paris! I can imagine the sailors from the Dutch East India Company coming into port here centuries ago. They may have enjoyed the brothels and then come to this church to beg forgiveness.

"There are women in the windows here, but we have women at home. We have nothing like this at home." I think my daughter understood because then she started to inspect the church with me.

As my daughter and I walked around the church, I thought: This is why we travel. Who knows what incredible thing awaits you around the next corner?

As the soft magenta sky turned dark grey, I thought about how fortunate I was to be able to take my family to this fantastic place that most people could only read about. My children were in their teens but not quite old enough to protest vacationing with their parents.

There had been difficulties in getting to Amsterdam. The first was flying in the economy section all night to get to Heathrow Airport and then having to eat beans for breakfast. There were smokers, Value-Added Taxes, and pickpockets. Of course, for me, there was the annoyance of being mistaken for a Japanese tourist. Yet, as we walked down the street, Oudekerksplien, back towards our hotel, I felt a moment of reflection and grace that I have so rarely experienced in life. The American Dream is being able to drive a foreign car and take your family for a vacation in Europe. I was the descendant of poor Japanese immigrants and yet here I was, living the American Dream.

Chapter 3

A Former Patient Sees Me and
Starts Crying

On Mother's Day morning, I drove to See's Candies at my local mall to purchase a gift for my wife. I didn't think I would have to wait in a long line as I would be getting there soon after opening. I was surprised to find that there were fifteen men in line ahead of me. I thought, "What is wrong with these men? Can't they think of anything more original than a box of chocolates? Also, why did they wait until the last minute to purchase their gift?" I wasn't even standing in front of the See's store. The line went to the mall entrance, and I was in front of the military recruitment store.

I promised myself that next year I would plan ahead. I had done some planning. I had driven to Costco the day before to purchase a See's gift card. I would thus be able to get a discount on a box of chocolates. It then occurred to me that I may have spent more money on gasoline than I would save with the gift certificate.

Finally, I got to the front of the line. The young saleswoman looked at me and asked, "Are you Dr. Matsumura?" At this point, I should mention that I am often recognized in public as I have delivered thousands of babies in my local community. Once, a patient recognized me from one hundred feet away. She ran towards me, calling out, "My doctor shops at the mall!" As she approached, I thought, "If we Asians all look alike, how does she know that it's me?" Anyway, at the See's store, I responded, "I am he." Immediately, her big brown eyes filled with tears. She looked me in the eye, then ran and hid in the back storage room.

I felt terrible. There were now twenty men in line behind me! There had been three saleswomen working as fast as they could, but now there were only two. One of the remaining saleswomen started passing out free sample chocolates as quickly as possible to prevent a riot.

More concerning to me was why did the saleswoman leave? Was she coming back? Had she left because she was overcome with happiness to see me? I decided that was not likely. She must have been a patient of mine in the past. Obviously, she had been distraught over my treatment. I didn't know if I should stay or leave. Before I could decide, she returned.

She told me that her name was Maria. Eight years earlier, she had come to this country from Mexico and could not speak any English. She had developed abdominal pain, lost consciousness, and had been taken to the Emergency Room in Vacaville. She was scared and concerned because she had no insurance. She told me that I had seen her in the Emergency Room and had treated her with respect and kindness, as had the entire staff. Lack of insurance had not become an issue. I had taken her to surgery, removed a ruptured tubal pregnancy, and sent her home later that same day. She said she had small scars on her abdomen now, but they were difficult to find. She said that I had removed a large amount of blood from her belly and had saved her life.

I told Maria that the surgery probably had saved her life, but I only did what any other gynecologist would have done in my place. I told her that I was glad that she had a good outcome. She wanted to embrace me, but the counter was too wide to reach across. She walked around the counter to hug me.

As she walked around, I glanced at the four customers immediately behind me. They were silent and had respectfully bowed their heads so that they would not appear to be eavesdropping on Maria's personal medical history.

It turned out that Maria was already in the first trimester of a new pregnancy. Soon she would be coming to see me for prenatal visits. At every appointment, she would bring me a box of chocolates. I can still remember what she brought me on St. Patrick's Day — a giant candy in a box that looked like an actual potato. The "dirt" on the outside of the potato was cocoa powder. I didn't care for the taste, but it was adorable.

As I drove home that Mother's Day, I looked at the bag holding my chocolates sitting in the passenger seat next to me. I could see that Maria had secretly stuffed my gift certificate back into my bag.

I then tried to remember the night I took care of Maria. That night, I probably complained to myself as I drove to the hospital that I should have been a dermatologist. (A common lament among obstetricians.) Maria may have spoken no English and had no insurance in her time of need, but her gratitude was more compensation than any insurance check. What a privilege it was to help a young woman who was struggling to make a new life for herself in this country.

Chapter 4

Culture Shock in Michigan

When my wife and I first became engaged, my wife's parents protested. They said that they feared we may have cultural differences that would be difficult to overcome. I could not see any cultural differences since both of us were only familiar with living in the United States. I thought their hesitation was simply due to racism (more on that later).

My wife and I brushed off her parents' concerns and married despite their misgivings. To my surprise, on my first visit to the state of Michigan, I found there were cultural differences.

I am a native of Mountain View, California, and my wife is from Flint, Michigan. Flint may not be so different from California today, but my wife lived her entire childhood there, pre-1975.

On our honeymoon, we went on a tour of the East Coast. I noticed my wife preferred an entrée of beef with a side order of potatoes, and occasionally, for variety, she would have an entrée of potatoes with a side order of beef. She also liked to order a dish that comes with several thinly cut slices of roast beef served on a piece of white bread and covered with gravy. My wife says it is called a hot beef sandwich. It is accompanied by mashed potatoes that are dispensed with an ice cream scoop. She was very content to eat this for both lunch and dinner — every day.

I soon became familiar with one of our famous American eatery chains that I will not mention by name, but it rhymes with Benny's. One of my favorite breakfasts there consisted of eggs and hash browns sitting on a thin bed of oil. The food was so greasy that once I swallowed it, I considered that there might not be any way to keep it from running all the way through. Even the bill comes a bit saturated with oil.

I like to eat something different every day. I like Japanese, Thai, Chinese, Vietnamese, Korean, Mexican, Indian, Italian, and basically all foods. The only food I am not fond of is British food, but I don't recall seeing many British restaurants in the United States. I would rather eat in an unfamiliar Thai restaurant than in a Benny's. My wife would not hear of it. I soon had the menu at Benny's memorized. For some reason, most of Benny's breakfast menu combinations end in the word "Slam." I picture the cook slamming the food items onto a plate and yelling, "Order up." For a long time, I was not sure if the chicken-fried steak was chicken or steak, but it didn't matter since it was fried. Either way, it was going to be good. It could be okra or eel; once it's fried, it's delicious.

My in-laws were aware of my fondness for Japanese food, so they took me to a Chinese restaurant (close enough) on my first trip to Flint, Michigan. I will never forget the name of the restaurant — Ivanhoe's. I speculate that the proprietor bought the restaurant, converted it to a Chinese restaurant, and didn't want to purchase a new sign. This was back in 1977. I believe the restaurant stayed in business until just a few years ago.

One of the plates we ordered may not be an authentic Chinese dish. It was sweet and sour chicken. I don't think any chickens were killed in making this dish, although there may be a chicken somewhere on crutches due to losing a leg. It consisted mainly of a sweet orange sauce over deep-fried battered chicken floating on a thin layer of oil. Maybe Benny's should add this to their menu.

My wife's family cooks a traditional potato soup they have been making for generations. It came from a Pennsylvania Dutch recipe and came to Michigan through my wife's ancestors who emigrated from Ohio. It consists of sliced potatoes, water, onions, and rivels. Rivels are little pieces of flour and egg mixture placed into the soup for flavor and texture. It is similar to store-bought pasta, but rivels are not formed into a shape. It gives you something to chew on to break up the monotony of just eating potatoes. The soup does not have cream or milk added, so it is very light. The soup is seasoned with a white spice that has been handed down for generations: salt. On the side, one has white bread with butter. The soup is paired with slightly chilled tap water. Although the meal is simple, it is surprisingly tasty.

I had two bowls and remarked how delicious it was, but I didn't find the meal very filling. I was in my early twenties then and had a large appetite. Looking back, I doubt that my in-laws approved when I finished off the meal with a bowl of Cheerios.

One day my in-laws told me I was in for a treat. We were going to go to the famous Michigan city of Frankenmuth. I asked, "What makes this city so famous?" My mother-in-law replied, "They have a store that sells Christmas decorations and another store that sells chicken dinners. We'll spend the whole afternoon there." "Whoa," I replied, "How have I never heard of this place?"

The Christmas store is more than a store. It's more like a theme park. The complex is called Bronner's, and I think it is the biggest Christmas store in the known world. I read that they will have as many as 50,000 shoppers on the weekend after Thanksgiving. They have over 300 decorated trees, 6,000 unique ornaments, and 500 nativity scenes. The showroom is longer than a football field.

I found a section of tree ornaments that said Merry Christmas in different languages. I had never seen such unique decorations in California. I found ornaments that said: Joyeux Noel, Frohliche Weihnachten, and Feliz Navidad. I was looking for one that would say Merry Christmas in Japanese. I finally found one and purchased it. I bought that big green ornament in 1977 and still have it today. It reads, "Merry Kurisumasu." Of course, that is not really a Japanese greeting. It is an adaptation of the English greeting.

Well, the fun didn't stop there. My in-laws knew I was not a fan of meat and potatoes, so while in Frankenmuth, we would be dining in a restaurant with far more exotic fare. The restaurant was called Zehnder's. It served fried chicken and mashed potatoes, but this was no KFC. The restaurant was huge. They can seat 1500 people simultaneously. In those days, dinner was only about $6 per person. The food was served family-style and was excellent.

Christmas comes just once a year, but not in the town of Frankenmuth. There, every day is Christmas. I thanked my in-laws for exposing me to this Bavarian Midwestern town.

The next day, we were back in Flint. The natives of Flint in the late twentieth century tended to eat at places with names like Wally's Supper Club and Bill Knapps. Wally's had a long buffet table that included meat and potatoes. For dessert, I found a wonderful green gelatin that had pineapple, mandarin oranges, and cottage cheese in it—a gastronomical delight. I was promptly told that in Michigan, it was not a dessert—it was a salad to be eaten with the main course. I quickly apologized and hoped the indigenous peoples did not notice I had it as a dessert.

It turned out that my in-laws were correct. There are cultural differences in the U.S., but they can be managed. It makes life more interesting to see how people live in other areas. Having done my obstetrical residency in the barrio of East Los Angeles (East L.A.), I can tell you there are more significant differences between East L.A. and West L.A. than between California and Michigan.

Chapter 5

A Jehovah's Witness Refuses Blood

One morning I saw my obstetrical partner, Dr. Goldman, in the hospital's doctor's lounge. The day before, she had caught me in the doctors' lounge surreptitiously eating bacon in a reading cubicle. "Why are you trying to hide the fact that you are eating bacon?" she asked. I told her not only was I a vegetarian, but my religion shunned the eating of pork. I had a lot of guilt and I was trying to hide it. I reminded her that her Jewish religion did not allow the eating of pork either — both our religions followed the same dietary restrictions proscribed in the book of Leviticus. She smiled and said, "I don't have a problem eating bacon or anything else for that matter."

Dr. Goldman looked different today. Her face showed she was distressed. She told me that while on call the night before, a teenage patient named Denise had to be admitted. Denise had abnormally heavy periods and her blood level had dropped to a dangerously low level. She was at the point where she could no longer walk or even stand without becoming lightheaded. Typically, we would give a patient like this young woman a blood transfusion. She was at risk of dying without blood, yet she refused it as she was a Jehovah's

Witness. Her mother was also a Jehovah's Witness and was encouraging her not to accept a transfusion. Dr. Goldman was very concerned that she was going to lose this patient. The patient's bleeding had slowed down with medical treatment but had not yet stopped.

I asked if I could talk to her patient. Dr. Goldman lit up and replied, "Oh please, would you?"

I have the utmost respect for other religions. I am certain this is because I want others to respect my religion. My parents raised me as a Seventh-day Adventist (SDA), and I attended SDA schools from grades one through medical school. That encompasses almost 20 years of Christian education. From grades one through eight, I attended Miramonte School. After that, I went to high school at Mountain View Academy. Then it was on to college and medical school at Loma Linda University.

I enjoyed my religion. It was great thinking that you were a member of God's family. We were not just a member of God's family—anyone can claim that. We were an exclusive group. We had the backstage passes. I wondered, "How can all the rest of the world be blind to the fact that we have the only true religion? Can they not see that if you read the Bible, we are the only Christians following God's teachings, starting with the fourth Commandment in Exodus 20?"

I found it disturbing (and still do) that we were required to show up for worship daily in college. Besides that, there were two mandatory services to attend: a late morning chapel service on Thursday and a church service on Sabbath (Saturday). In the 1970s, I can clearly remember seeing my Resident Assistant (RA) standing on the steps at the front of the chapel and dictating my name into a portable plastic reel-to-reel tape recorder. He would later return to the dorm and go over his checklist of absentee students. One could only have a limited number of absences. I no longer remember what the punishment was for missing too many religious services. I don't know if this practice is still in force today, but I hope not.

Although I don't remember the consequences of breaking some rules at college, there is one that I remember clearly. I had a friend whose boyfriend came to visit her. He spent the night in her dorm room, sleeping on the floor. Her roommate was present. Nevertheless, she was still expelled. The only time men were allowed in the women's dorm in the 1970s was on moving-in day.

I recently learned that things were just as restrictive at another SDA college that my sister Lynda attended. She attended Pacific Union College in Northern California. She had a friend named Takashi from Japan who was not fluent in English. Lynda would help him do his homework at the house she was staying at. If he had a reading assignment, first she would have to translate the pages and then help him write his report, which was very time-consuming. He would often not make it back to his dorm by the 10 pm curfew. Lynda would call the dorm to explain why he would be late getting in, but there were a limited number of excuses one could have. One night she called the dorm to explain, but the monitor said that Takashi had used up all of his excuses and now the dean of the dorm would have to notify Takashi's parents. Lynda became indignant. She said, "You do know Takashi is 30 years old and English is not his first language, right?" She then told the monitor to be sure the dean was aware of the time difference in Japan where Takashi's parents lived and added, "By the way, they don't speak English." The monitor insisted the parents would still have to be notified. Lynda replied, "Knock yourself out." Takashi's parents were never notified. Well, I digress, but suffice it to say that I received more than my share of an exclusive and peculiar Christian education.

After my formal education, I did my OB/GYN residency at an SDA medical center in Southern California.

My father was the first Japanese in the United States to be born into an SDA family. I was reminded of this many times by Mr. Watanabe, a patriarch in our church. One could say that I have been indoctrinated. Even though I no longer attend church, I cannot completely remove myself from my religion after that many years.

As a teenager, I'd get a job every summer to earn money. I'd make it clear to my potential employer that I could not work on the Sabbath (Saturdays). Fortunately, this was never a hindrance to my gaining employment.

With this profoundly religious background, how could I not respect Jehovah's Witnesses and their devout beliefs—even though I was no longer a believer?

I studied the patient's chart before entering her room. Denise was thin and pale. Rather than having a rosy hue to her face, her skin looked yellow. She was scared, but oriented. Her mother was the only other person with her. I said to Denise's mother, "Hi Mrs. Gunderson, I am Dr. Goldman's partner, Dr. Matsumura. Would it be okay with you if I talked to Denise about her bleeding?"

Mrs. Gunderson replied, "Are you going to try to talk her into accepting a blood transfusion?"

I responded, "I think a blood transfusion is very much indicated and could be lifesaving at this point, but Denise can certainly refuse it."

"Ok," said Mrs. Gunderson, "but you should know that we are Jehovah's Witnesses, and we do not accept blood or blood products."

I told them I also had a strong religious background. I then explained it was common for patients to initially refuse blood out of respect for their devout Jehovah's Witness family members that accompanied them to the hospital.

I said, "Denise, at the end of our discussion, I will ask you: 'If you have to choose between receiving a blood transfusion and dying, would you prefer to die? You have decision-making capacity and have the right to self-determination.'"

I continued, "Denise, this country was founded by people that left Europe so they could practice their religion as they saw fit. About half of them died the first year trying to establish a foothold in this country. Ultimately, we will honor your wishes."

I then asked Denise if I could speak with her privately to determine her true feelings about blood transfusion and make certain she was not under any duress from her family to refuse or accept blood, based on their beliefs. Denise replied, "I would be more comfortable if you spoke to both my mother and me together."

Through the years, I have learned that there is considerable variation in what individuals will and will not accept. Some will take certain blood components. Some Jehovah's Witnesses will take their own blood back through a cell-saver device used in surgery (not relevant in this case). It was our job to determine exactly what Denise would find acceptable. I was not supposed to engage the patient in debate. For one thing, we physicians are the patient's advocates, and we don't want to place ourselves in an adversarial position with the patient. Nevertheless, I soon found myself getting into a religious discussion.

I told Denise that this was her mother's religion and not necessarily hers as far as I could tell. Denise drank alcohol and was sexually active with her boyfriend—two activities that were frowned upon by her religion and many others. I told her there would be plenty of time to decide if she wanted to accept her mother's religion as her own, but she did not have to make that decision today.

I asked Denise if she knew why Jehovah's Witnesses did not accept blood. She said it was because there were texts in the Bible that said, "Life is in the blood." I asked her if she knew the exact texts. She said she did not. I then told her, "I don't know either, but in Genesis, it says that after the flood, God told Noah and his family that they could add meat to their diets, but they were instructed not to eat the blood."

I told Denise, "Since blood transfusions were not possible in those days, I don't think they were addressing what should be done if one needed a blood transfusion."

Mrs. Gunderson interjected: "We don't think the Bible was trying to address blood transfusions. The blood is life. We believe the blood is too sacred to be taken from one person and given to another."

I told her, "I can respect that point of view. My religion forbids the eating of shellfish and pork; thus, I have gone almost my entire life not eating either, although I don't think a loving God would hold it against me if I needed to eat those things to survive."

I asked Denise if she thought homosexuality was okay. She said she thought it was. I told her I did not always think so, but now I felt as she did. I asked her if she knew what the Bible had to say about homosexuality. She said that she knew it was not acceptable in the Bible. I told her that the book of Leviticus says that if a man lies with another man, as he would with a woman, both men should be put to death.

I then changed the subject, "Denise, do you know what the Bible says about slavery?" She replied, "No, I don't know."

"In Leviticus, it says that you can buy male and female slaves from nations around you or you can buy slaves from foreigners living in your land, and they can be your property. Your sons can inherit your slaves. In Colossians, slaves are told to 'Obey your earthly masters … with sincerity of heart and fear of the Lord.' During the Civil War, Southerners would quote these texts to justify the institution of slavery. It might have prevented a lot of controversies if the Bible had said, 'Slavery needs to be abolished,' but it didn't."

I could feel myself tensing up. I told myself not to let this turn into an argumentative discussion or we would both dig deeper into our positions. I decided to lighten up the conversation.

I then said, "I think of religion as a menu. You choose what you like and leave the rest. My son and daughter like to eat at poke bowl restaurants when they are in Hawaii."

"You digress a lot, don't you?" Mrs. Gunderson smiled and relaxed a bit.

"I...I...yes."

"What is poke?" Denise asked.

"Poke is often a raw Ahi tuna that has been marinated in something like soy sauce."

"Interesting, that sounds good." As the conversation digressed, Denise also started to relax.

"Well, for me, it is a bit slimy, but anyway, one restaurant they frequent asks you to make some choices. They ask you to choose a base: brown or white rice, a protein: tuna, or tofu; and third, they ask you to choose your sides: imitation crab, avocado, etc. Let's call it the trinity of Poke food prep."

"Religion is similar. You choose a God, then religion, and finally a denomination. The God you choose may vary depending on whether you are a Jew, Christian, Muslim, etc."

"Which religion did you choose?" Denise asked.

"I took the easy route, as you did, which was to take on the religion of my parents. It was a no-brainer. My parents were Seventh-day Adventists, as that was the religion of their parents. As children, we have no choice but to take on the religion of our parents. We can change it as we get older, but few do."

Denise asked, "Do you still go to church?"

"I do not, although I have to say that my religion got me through some challenging times in my younger life."

Mrs. Gunderson then said, "I cannot imagine never seeing my deceased parents again. I have to believe there is something more waiting for us."

"Are you saying that you believe in Heaven because you don't like the alternative of there not being an afterlife?"

"No, I believe God has something more in store for us for other reasons, too." Mrs. Gunderson stiffened up with indignation.

"If you believe in religion because it gives you comfort and peace of mind, who am I to try to take that away from you? When I was a believer, I also found peace in leaving everything in God's hands, but once I realized I was a Seventh-day Adventist because that was the religion my parents gave me, it made me ask questions. What if I had been born in Japan? I don't know the most popular religion in Japan, but I'm guessing it's not Christianity. It would have been different if my parents had required me to study all the major religions and then choose the one that made the most sense. That I could respect.

"As I got older, I began to question things like, why would God allow over fifty million people to die in World War II? Every family in Europe knew loss. Some families were wiped out. Why is it God's will to have a child born with profound cerebral palsy who grows up to be an adult with very little quality of life? What is God's plan for that person and his family? Some missionaries train for years to be able to spread the Word of God. They then pray for God's protection but are killed in the mission field. What was God's plan for them and for those they were going to help?

"I was born in the U.S., so I was born a Christian. I was born into God's only true religion. But wait, everyone thinks they are born into God's only true religion. If you were born in India, you are a Hindu. If you were born in an Arab nation, you are a Muslim. If you were born in Mexico, you are Catholic. We take on the religion of our country and our parents. If you live in Limerick, Ireland, you are a Catholic, and everyone in your family is as well. You can hardly say the word Irish without adding Catholic. It works out well until you marry a Protestant and then your family disowns you.

"It reminds me of a *Family Guy* cartoon. Baby Stewie is taken to the mall and is pleasantly surprised to find Santa there. He says, 'Of all the malls in the world, Santa chooses to come to this one. What are the odds?' I'll tell you what the odds are: They are one hundred percent! Every mall has a Santa. And what are the odds that you will be born into God's only true religion? They are one hundred percent.

"Over time, however, children stop believing in Santa. Believing in Santa tapers off significantly by age eight or nine. Even after children figure out that there is no Santa, they play along for a while. Why ruin a good thing, right? Children don't have to be told by an older child that Santa doesn't exist. As children get older, they develop a rough sense of how many children there are in the world and how many toys will fit into a single flying sleigh. The whole concept falls apart."

One would think that children would then learn to be skeptical, realize that parents don't always tell the truth when it comes to the supernatural. That doesn't happen as children continue to believe that their parents chose God's true religion for them.

"I think there are about twenty million Seventh-day Adventists in the world. I am going to tell you something that not even one of those Adventists believes, but I think you will agree with me—The SDA church is not God's one true religion. I do not believe your religion is the only true religion either. Religion is not truth. Religion is just an organization that is seeking God's truths."

"Doctor, may I interrupt you?" Denise said. "I want to get that blood transfusion."

Her statement startled me. I then said, "Denise, honestly, that was my goal when I walked into your room, and at this point, I should just shut up, but at the risk of you changing your mind, I want to give you full disclosure. I don't know the correct answers to this or any other religious questions. I am just putting forth my best guesses. The longer I live, the more questions I have. When I was young, I thought I knew the answers. Now I don't.

"I have only known you for a few minutes, but I will tell you what I do know for sure. I know you are a beautiful person both inside and out. I know that your mother loves you more than you will ever know unless you have children of your own. I think that a loving God would want you to have a fulfilling life and not just die as a teen."

Denise's mother broke down and sobbed with her face in her hands. I asked her if she was upset with me as her daughter was now willing to accept blood. She said, "No, I am just so relieved that my daughter is not going to die."

Denise's mother explained that although she believed her daughter should not accept blood, she also believed if her daughter died now, she might not see her again. She then said, "Although you and I disagree when it comes to religion, I want to thank you for caring enough to talk to Denise even though she is not your patient."

After talking with Denise and her mother, I felt spent. There was so much riding on that discussion. I realized that it could have just as easily gone the other way, but those are the uncertainties of being a physician. I knew I was only supposed to discuss the risks, benefits, and alternatives of blood transfusion with Denise and determine what she wanted. It was not my role to engage her in religious debate. I had overstepped my bounds. I brought my personal views into the discussion. Had I applied inappropriate pressure to get Denise to accept blood? When I told Denise that I didn't think this was her religion but was her mother's — I should have left it at that and then let her make her decision.

I often find myself second-guessing my decisions in medicine, wondering if I could have done better. I've had a lot of formal training in managing patients, yet sometimes I feel as though I'm just winging it. I wonder if other physicians second-guess themselves as much as I did.

Well, at least Denise will live to see another day. That's important, right? I'll be happy with that and move on to my next patient.

Chapter 6

Talking To God

If I ever meet God in Heaven, I am going to have a lot of questions. Our conversation could go like this:

Dr. M: God, you've answered many questions for me today, but I have just one more question.

God: Well, Dr. Matsumura, I am here to help.

Dr. M: Oh please God, call me Gary.

God: Okay, what is your question?

Dr. M: What was your true religion on Earth?

God: Well, let's see. I guess the Mormons were the closest.

Dr. M: I think they prefer to be called members of The Church of Jesus Christ of Latter-Day Saints.

God: Yeah, let's call them Mormons. What do you know about that religion?

Dr. M: Well, my religion has some similarities to that religion. Both groups don't smoke, nor do they drink alcohol or coffee. I know that Joseph Smith prayed to God—I mean to you—to ask which religion to join, and you supposedly said that none of the religions were your true religion, so he should start a brand new faith. An angel brought gold plates with Egyptian writing on them to Smith. He translated these plates with unique spectacles. He lost the original plates, and

I'm guessing the glasses too, but the translated plates became the *Book of Mormon*. The book tells of a man named Lehi who left Jerusalem by boat in 589 BC, way before Columbus, and came to North America. There he converted the Native Americans to Christianity. I believe you told Joseph Smith to have more than one wife. There was pressure from the government to give that up, so they did. I may have some details wrong, but that is what I remember. It always seemed like an unbelievable story to me.

God: Well, to hear you tell it, it does sound made up, but no, that was my true religion.

Dr. M: I should not have made so many jokes about Joseph Smith misplacing the gold plates.

God: No, and do you remember what you said when two Mormons showed up at your front door in shirt sleeves?

Dr. M: No.

God: Well, you said, "*Konichiwa*." You pretended to speak only Japanese.

Dr. M: Ha, you have to admit that was kind of funny.

God: Yeah, that was kinda funny.

Dr. M: Wow, I just remembered something. I had a neonatologist friend who is a Mormon, but I never thought he was a member of the one true religion. Who knew?

God: I did.

I have good friends who are Mormons, but I hope that I do not find out someday that they are members of the only true religion. If they are, then I should not have been making fun of their strange beliefs, especially since my faith has equally absurd views. There are thousands of religions in the world. I think I am safe.

Chapter 7

Boba Tea

In 2004, I worked as an OB Hospitalist at Washington Hospital in Fremont, California. An OB Hospitalist's duties include caring for obstetrical patients who do not have a doctor and helping regular staff doctors with cesareans and emergencies. The shifts would last twenty-four hours. When on duty, I was never supposed to be far from the obstetrical floor in case of an emergency. My fellow OB Hospitalists wanted to ask if we could leave the hospital campus to eat in the local restaurants. I insisted that they not ask, as I was afraid the answer would be no. I soon had visited every restaurant within a few blocks of the hospital. I found no better Indian or Afghan food in the San Francisco Bay Area than in Fremont.

It was at this time that I discovered a refreshing beverage. It was a new drink at the time but is found commonly now. It goes by various names: bubble tea, pearl tea, boba tea, and I am sure there are other names for it. It can be made as a smoothie or as a tea. I was eating at my favorite Chinese restaurant in Fremont when the owner brought me a free sample of this Taiwanese fruit smoothie. The flavor was honeydew. It looked like the green Shamrock milkshake that McDonald's sells on

St. Patrick's Day. I noticed immediately that this drink was unusual. It had black balls on the bottom the size of gumballs and came with a very wide caliber straw so you could suck up those big balls. It was tea with dumplings.

I am told that the term "bubble" is an Anglicized imitative word derived from the Taiwanese word boba, which means "large breasts" and is slang for the large, chewy, black tapioca balls added to the drink.

The owner had a poster on the wall that advertised this particular beverage. It had a picture of the same green drink I was having with the caption: "Let Me Crazy." I think the caption meant: "Let me be crazy by allowing me to have this interesting drink."

It was the most refreshing drink I had ever tasted! This was amazing as I don't care that much for honeydew. As I would suck on the wide straw, with every sip, one or two of these giant, rubbery tapioca balls would be deposited into my mouth. The balls don't have to be black, but the black color allows one to quickly see how many balls are left at the bottom of your drink.

At first, I thought this was strange. How often do you chew your drink? It isn't the tapioca balls that make the drink so good. Sometimes I will order the drink without the balls if I am not ordering in a place that specializes in boba drinks. There is nothing worse than soggy balls. You want your balls fresh and firm, as you would your pasta.

Every time I returned to this restaurant, I would order the same drink. Although it comes in many flavors, I only ordered honeydew. I was concerned that if I asked for any other flavor, I would be disappointed.

After my discovery, I would, on occasion, offer to buy boba teas for the entire floor of excellent OB nurses. I would ask which flavor they would like. There were over thirty flavors to choose from, but almost all the Filipina nurses would ask for avocado. It turned out this restaurant made boba teas with fresh avocado. I thought they would have asked for taro, peach, mango, or some other popular flavor. "You want a guacamole milkshake?" I asked. They found it to be delicious. I wasn't willing to try it.

I immediately wanted to share my discovery with my family and friends. I e-mailed my son, who was a student at U.C. Davis at the time. He told me he had been drinking bubble pearl teas for some time. He said they were more popular than Chai tea in Davis.

It turned out that most of my other Asian relatives and friends were also already familiar with this drink. It seemed I was the only one who was making this latent discovery. I felt somewhat inadequate as an Asian, not for the first time.

I have a Caucasian friend who thinks she is Asian. Her name is Barbara. She dresses up in a red Asian silk dress. She looks like she could be working for an evil bald villain who pets a hairless cat. Her hair is up in a bun held together with chopsticks. She can speak Japanese, and of course, she is familiar with Asian foods. I asked her if she was familiar with the pearl tea drink. She said, "Of course, this drink is trendy in and out of the Asian community. You are a disgrace to your heritage. You are a banana." That is a derogatory term to denote someone who is yellow on the outside and white on the inside. I was familiar with the expression. There is also a term for her—a hard-boiled egg.

Chapter 8

Cesarean Section

My First Cesarean

The first cesarean I observed in my residency was compelling. I didn't understand how the surgeon could tell what layer of tissue he was working on—it all looked the same. Before long, it was time for me to do my first C-section. By then, I had assisted in enough of them to know I could do the job.

The patient was given her spinal anesthetic. She was cleaned and draped so only her abdomen was showing. The patient's face was behind the drapes, so she could not see us or the surgery. My assistant was Dr. Stevens. He was a very enthusiastic intern. He loved medicine, and he loved life. He eventually changed his residency from obstetrics to surgery and then to emergency medicine. He changed residencies so many times that I don't know what he ultimately ended up doing. Anyway, Dr. Stevens was very excited that this was the first cesarean where I was the primary surgeon and not the assistant.

I was about to make the initial incision when Dr. Stevens announced to the operating room staff: "This is to be Dr. Matsumura's first C-section!" I was shocked. Dr. Stevens had forgotten that the patient was having her surgery while fully awake. I frantically pointed toward the patient's head, indicating that the patient could hear what he was saying. He immediately got the message and became very quiet. I could see that he had a sheepish grin on his face even though he had his mask on.

This patient spoke Spanish, as did most of our patients in East Los Angeles. That did not mean that the patient didn't speak or understand English. Once, we had a patient in labor who would cry out with every contraction: "Ay, ay, ay, ay!" She only spoke Spanish, or so we thought. The intern had been having a little fun with her. He had repeatedly said, "I'm sorry, but we don't have an eye doctor here." After the delivery, he went back to her and asked, "Como estas?" She replied, "I am doing well. I feel so much better, thanks." It turned out that she could speak perfect English. He was very embarrassed and apologized.

Maternal Death

I was only into the second week of my OB residency in East Los Angeles when we had a maternal death. I still remember the attending surgeon was Dr. Robb. We were doing a cesarean section when the anesthesiologist announced that the patient's condition had suddenly deteriorated. I remember that the patient's blood was no longer red but more of a blue color. That patient died instantly from an amniotic fluid embolism. Dr. Robb started doing CPR. My jaw dropped as I saw what was unfolding around me. Fluid from the patient's bag of water had escaped into her bloodstream and had given her a total cardio-respiratory collapse. My intern and friend, Dr. Bruce, started to rethink his choice of going into obstetrics that day. The patient's twins both survived. They would be adults now. The patient's husband was very brave and showed very little emotion. He had to be in a state of shock. He thanked us for doing our best.

The husband later tried to sue us because of the maternal death. An autopsy showed fetal skin cells in the mother's lungs, showing that it truly was a case of amniotic fluid embolism and therefore, not our fault. Amniotic fluid embolism is rare and often fatal. It is not preventable.

I learned a lot that day. I learned that not all obstetrical outcomes were favorable. I learned that although you are your patient's advocate, things can change quickly when things don't go well. The patient, or in this case her family, can become your adversary.

Performing a Cesarean in the Emergency Room (E.R.)

There was a popular television show called *ER* some years ago. I didn't care to watch it, as I found watching that show to be somewhat stressful. I found myself trying to come up with diagnoses and treatments. It reminded me too much of work. Medical shows are not generally realistic. I have enjoyed *House, Grey's Anatomy, Doc Martin, and Scrubs*, but I am careful not to take the shows too seriously.

The point is to just be entertained. No one in the room watching with you wants to hear you keep saying, "That would never happen." Instead of rolling your eyes, you just have to roll with it as if you are watching a time travel movie. *ER* was well written and interesting. The cast members were attractive. From watching the show, one could get the impression that the E.R. is an exciting and interesting place to work and that many of the staff are intimately involved. That has not been my experience. Having worked in the E.R., my preference would be to work in the kitchen scrubbing pots and pans. I found the E.R. to be full of people that didn't need emergency treatment. They just didn't have a regular doctor to visit as they didn't have health insurance. Many are alcoholics or are suffering from some other addiction. Some come in so often they are known as "frequent flyers." Of course, E.R. physicians may not feel as I do.

Anyway, one morning a patient came into my office for her routine prenatal visit. She was obviously very distressed. She was almost due, so you can imagine her concern when she was watching the show *ER* the night before and to her amazement, they had a maternal death. Before I go on, I must say that maternal death is the thing that I fear the most in medicine, although, for some reason, I never verbalize that fear. Death may occur commonly in other specialties of medicine, but in obstetrics, maternal death is rare.

A trauma surgeon told me that trauma surgery on a pregnant woman is the most stressful of surgeries. First of all, you have to worry about two patients. The other issue is that families expect the worst with trauma, and trauma patients do die. For some reason, no one expects or is prepared for a pregnant woman to die. The patient is young and everyone is expecting a positive outcome. They are not supposed to die.

I asked my patient to describe to me what had happened in the *ER* episode she had watched. She said that the E.R. had a pregnant patient come in and was seen by Dr. Green. I responded, "Ah, he is a top gun physician." The patient had a little protein in her urine. Dr. Green thought this indicated a urinary infection, so he prescribed an antibiotic and sent her home. She later returned to the E.R. in florid toxemia, also known as preeclampsia. (Preeclampsia is a disease of the latter part of pregnancy where the woman has elevated blood pressure and protein in the urine.) Dr. Green realized his mistake and felt that it was his fault that the diagnosis wasn't made sooner before the disease became out of control. (Apparently, Dr. Green was not so much a nerd as one of his earlier films indicated, or he would have made the diagnosis on her first visit.)

Dr. Green tried to get the OB department to take the patient, but they were full at that time. He decided he had to do an emergency C-section in the E.R. or the patient would continue to deteriorate. He performed the cesarean, trying to remember from his intern days how to perform the procedure. After starting the cesarean, he remembered there was something about making a bladder flap. That part about the bladder flap was put in for the benefit of us OB/GYNs. He successfully delivered a healthy baby, but it was too late for the mother. She died from preeclampsia. The last scene was when Dr. Green had to tell the husband that his baby was fine, but they couldn't save his wife. Dr. Green took the husband into a private room. The camera did not enter the room, but the room had glass windows, so, although one could not hear the dialog, Dr. Green could be seen explaining the situation to the husband. One cannot imagine a more difficult conversation. Although both Dr. Green and the husband were standing, the husband collapsed his face into his own hands on hearing the news. The scene was very poignant.

I told the patient that this must have been an exceptionally moving show for her to watch while she was approaching the time of her own delivery. I then asked her in a quiet and respectful voice, "Do you know why that patient died in the E.R.?" "No," she replied.

I went on, "She died because she was operated on by an actor." The patient looked at me with confusion at first and then started to smile as she got the point. "The story is made up, isn't it?" she responded.

I replied, "It is totally fictional and the OB unit is never closed. If a busload of pregnant women gets into a motor vehicle accident, we will take all of them even if we have to put patients in the hallway and place portable partitions between them."

"Furthermore," I continued, "in the real world, if a pregnant patient trips and breaks her big toe, she is sent up to the labor and delivery suite from the E.R. to be certain that her baby is stable before they will even do an X-ray of her toe."

The Actual Cesarean Procedure

Before doing a cesarean, the doctor explains the risks, benefits, and alternatives of the procedure as he would before any procedure. There are cases where the mother's bag of water is broken. She has a uterine infection and is exhausted after being in labor for multiple days, yet she is still not making progress. In this case, and many others, there really isn't any alternative to a cesarean.

After the consent is signed, the patient is given an anesthetic. With few exceptions, the patient is given an anesthetic in her back instead of a general anesthetic where she would be put to sleep. This is safer for mom and baby. The baby ends up not getting any anesthesia. It also allows the partner and patient to witness the baby's first cry as a couple.

Skin: First, a careful incision is made in the skin. In lay terms, this incision is called a bikini cut instead of a vertical incision that goes from the belly button to the pubic hairline. One must be careful to make the scar as symmetrical as possible because this is the only part of the surgery that the patient sees. Many patients tell me that their previous obstetrician was an excellent doctor because they are pleased with how their scar looks.

When we do a cesarean, we incise each layer of the abdomen.

Once a patient came back to me for her post-cesarean visit and complained that I had cut her bikini incision too high and that it showed when she wore a bikini. It bothered me that she was not satisfied with her scar, so I asked her at the following visit if the scar really did show. She replied, "Of course not. I was just giving you a hard time. Do you think I wear my bikini so low that my muff is hanging out? Besides, after having a baby, very few of us ever wear a bikini again." I was relieved. Nowadays, this would not be a problem because many women have shaved off their "muff."

Fat: After incising the skin, the obstetrician cuts through the fat. This is called adipose tissue, but it is really just fat. One would think they could just call it that. This layer can be thin or over eight inches thick in women who weigh over 400 pounds. For a woman who is morbidly obese, I may get some four-inch duct tape and lift her tummy fat toward the head of the table. The tape looks like wide suspenders going from the lower abdomen over her shoulders to the head of the table. This allows me to do my bikini cut without going through so much fat. With the help of the tape, some women's fat layer may be the same thickness as a thin patient's in the area of the bikini cut.

It was difficult to weigh women who weighed over 400 pounds in the old days because doctors' scales didn't go that high. When I was a medical student, I once had a Samoan patient that said she was weighed at the truck stop. I don't know if that meant she was weighed by herself or if she had her car weighed with and without her in it.

I once made a mistake while doing a cesarean on a woman who weighed more than 400 pounds. I was doing a repeat cesarean and made my incision in the old vertical scar of her previous cesarean section. Her old scar started at her belly button and went down vertically to her pubic bone. Apparently, she had gained considerable weight since her previous cesarean. I cut deeper and deeper into the fat but never came to anything but more fat, so I kept cutting. I finally realized that if I kept cutting, I would come out the other side of her skin without ever encountering the uterus and the baby.

As it turned out, I was cutting into her panniculus, that is, her tummy roll, which she wore down towards her knees like an apron. Realizing my mistake, I extended my incision above her belly button and soon found her uterus. The patient ultimately healed well without any complications. I later had to explain my mistake when telling her why her new incision was longer than her old one. She told me not to worry about it. She was just happy that her baby was healthy.

Muscle: The next step in doing a cesarean involves dividing the rectus muscle. This is the muscle that is sometimes described as a six-pack when it is well-defined. One can simply divide this muscle with your fingers without necessarily cutting into it. Some surgeons suture this layer back together on the way out so that the patient doesn't have a big bulge there when she does sit-ups.

Peritoneum: This is the thin final layer that is cut through to enter the abdominal cavity. Some doctors no longer close this layer on the way out because it closes very quickly by itself. I always close it, as I believe it prevents excessive scar tissue. Doctors tell me that I am wrong. I ignore them.

Bladder: Generally, at this point, we "make a bladder flap," that is, we take the bladder down away from the uterus, giving us a greater margin of safety as we don't want to be near the bladder when we make the uterine incision. Some doctors consider this an unnecessary step.

Uterus: Finally, we are at the uterus. We now take a scalpel and enter the uterus to remove the baby.

Unfortunately, one can easily nick the baby's face at this point because the baby is often pressed up against the other side of the uterine wall. You can imagine trying to use a scalpel to cut through a Band-Aid without cutting the skin below it. We all have our little tricks to avoid cutting the baby's face. For instance, as I realize I am almost through the full thickness of the uterus, I may put down the scalpel and enter the uterus with my blunt finger.

I recall a case many years ago when my partner and I were going to Vallejo to start practicing at the hospital there. That hospital did not enjoy a good reputation at that time (although it does now). Since we were coming from a better-known hospital in Fairfield, we thought we were hot stuff walking through their corridors. As I made the incision through the uterus, I made a small nick on the baby's face. Well, so much for thinking we were hotshots. Fortunately, the baby's face healed without a scar (which is almost always the case). I later explained to the patient what had happened. She was cheerful and very forgiving. I was so embarrassed that I have not made that mistake since. Cesareans go rather quickly, but at that point in the surgery, at least for me, the procedure almost stops so that I can enter the uterus carefully.

In an emergency, a baby can be delivered by cesarean in about a minute from the time of the skin incision. One only needs a scalpel to get the baby out. When we practice doing emergency cesareans on a simulator dummy, I always tell my assistant to keep her fingers out of the way of my scalpel. Generally, the entire case takes about an hour. Most of that time is spent putting the mother back together. I know an obstetrician who routinely does the entire cesarean in about ten minutes. I feel we should do a personnel finger count after those cases. I'm not sure what the rush is. Maybe that doctor thinks that there is less time for the germs to jump in when you do a cesarean that rapidly.

Mother Does Her Own Cesarean

A cesarean is a delicate and exact surgery that requires considerable skill to perform — or so I thought. I read in a newspaper years ago about a woman in Mexico who performed a cesarean on herself. The woman was forty years old. She was having her ninth child. Labor was not going well, and she had previously lost a child in childbirth.

She did not have running water or electricity. She drank three shots of hard liquor to numb herself somewhat. She then performed a cesarean on herself with a kitchen knife and delivered a healthy son. I think she must have made a vertical incision on the abdomen.

Fortunately, she did not bleed excessively. Before she lost consciousness, she called a nurse who came over and sewed her together with an ordinary needle and thread. She then took an eight-hour car ride to the nearest hospital in Oaxaca. What incredible dedication a woman can have to save her unborn child.

Chapter 9

Southern Accents

We have a shortage of nurses in our local hospital. It has been this way for as long as I can remember. To provide our patients with an adequate supply of nursing care, we will sometimes import nurses from other parts of the country. We get a lot of them from the South.

There is something very genuine about people with a Southern accent. The Southern accent is very relaxed, folksy, and not pretentious. At first, I was concerned that some of these nurses from the South might not like me, as I am a minority. They turned out to be the friendliest nurses I have ever met. After they leave, they stay in contact with you.

In Alabama, the Southern drawl has a beautiful twang, but it can be difficult to decipher.

When we got our first batch of Southern nurses, I had a difficult time understanding them. We had one nurse from Alabama named Delane. One day she said to me, "Aam glad you're here now 'cause aah was just fixin' to call you. Yore patient Missus Bay-yell is hav'in premature contractions ag'in." I said, "I don't have a patient by that name." She said, "Yes, you do, you bin tak'in care of Missus Bay-yell all week. Not wanting to offend Delane, I asked, "How do you spell Bay-yel?" She replied, "B-e-l-l." "Oh," I said, "that Mrs. Bay-yel."

Later, Delane told me that the other nurses had been talking about me. She said, "They bin talkin 'bout choo; not me, they-yem."

I am aware of a midwife who was talking to a pregnant patient from the South. The patient had pain when she sat down. She tried to explain this to the midwife, but she pronounced sit as "see-yit." She would say, "It hurts when aah see-yit." The midwife then asked, "It hurts when you see what?" "It hurts when aah see-yit." "When you see what?" "It hurts when aah see-yit on a chair." "When you see what on a chair?"

Finally, the patient showed her that it hurt when she sat down.

We use a translating service in our obstetrical unit. It is a telephone that lets you have a mini-conference call as it has two hand pieces on it. You can call a number and be provided with an interpreter in almost any language you can think of. I've thought about calling this service and asking if anyone there speaks Southern.

Chapter 10

Man Clogs

One day I noticed my obstetrician partner, Dr. Fredericks, was wearing clogs. They looked very comfortable, and I've always preferred shoes that didn't have to be laced up. When I would be on call in the hospital, I would frequently have to get out of bed several times per night. That necessitated me putting on and taking off my shoes over and over. Clogs would be the next best thing to wearing slippers.

I was not used to seeing men wearing clogs. I had a roommate in the 1970s who wore clogs, but he was Scandinavian.

I decided to go to the internet to see if I could find clogs that didn't look like clogs. I didn't know what I was really looking for. Did I really think I could find clogs disguised as wingtips? On the internet, I found that there are support groups for men who want to wear clogs but need some encouragement.

I decided I would start with beginner clogs. I was not secure enough to buy the clogs with the open heel. Even gay men aren't ready for that.

I went to the local shoe store in my mall on a Tuesday morning, knowing there wouldn't be many people there. I found some Dansko brand clogs in some attractive colors. They came in dark green, oxblood (or cordovan), navy blue, etc. I thought it was a bit strange that the size that fit me was a size 41. I usually only wear a size 8. The salesman there tried to be helpful and directed me to the men's section.

In the men's section, I noticed that the clogs only came in black. By now, I had my heart set on the oxblood clogs. They were a vibrant, dark burgundy color, and human blood would not stain them. I didn't think that they looked feminine at all. I went back to the "other" section and decided to make my purchase. I told the salesman that I was buying the clogs for a friend.

"I see," he replied. "Apparently, you and your friend wear the same size shoe."

"That's right," I replied. I watched him to make sure he didn't wink. If he had, I would have hit him with my shoulder bag.

I originally was only going to wear my clogs at work when I was wearing my scrubs. That would be socially acceptable.

I soon became very comfortable with my new clogs. I would get home from a long day at work and would slip out of my clogs while I was still walking — how efficient. My wife quickly put an end to that because she would find them in the middle of our entryway. If I needed to go outside to feed the cats or take out the garbage, I didn't have to bother putting on traditional shoes anymore.

Over time, I found myself wearing my clogs more and my regular shoes less. I guess what happened next was inevitable. I accidentally wore my clogs out to dinner. There they were, and I slipped them on as I had done so many times previously when I was going to the hospital. My son, seeing my clogs asked, "Dad, aren't those shoes a little effeminate?"

"Aren't you a little rude?" I replied.

I was a bit surprised to hear this coming from my son Eric. When we go out to a nice restaurant, he always asks how he should dress, even though he is an adult with children of his own. If he doesn't, his mother will be sure to ask, "You don't plan to go out like that, do you?" I always recommend that he wear "good school clothes." He thinks that means he should wear clean shorts to go with his all-occasion flip-flops.

My wife, Kathy, also likes to give my daughter, Kristen, advice on how to dress when going out. Once, we were in Reno, Nevada, to attend my uncle's funeral. The only shoes my daughter had brought were black flip-flops. Kathy and Kristen had a "discussion" about that.

Well, because of my son's relaxed attitude, I didn't think that he would have even noticed my clogs. My son explained that contrary to popular belief, young people do have a dress code. He went on, "Yes, we might wear flip-flops to a fancy restaurant, but we wouldn't wear them with socks."

The nurses in the labor and delivery suite complimented me on my choice of clogs. They reassured me that I had chosen one of the better brands and could now enjoy many years of podiatric comfort. Nurse Lee would comment with a smile, "Oh, I see you are wearing your man clogs." Somehow this sounded like something my son would say. Could she possibly be making fun of me, or was I being overly sensitive? I decided I didn't care. At this point, they were too comfortable to give up.

I found that nurses loved to talk about my clogs and compare them to their own. They are very supportive of men wearing clogs. They think a man is more sensitive and accepting if he is willing to open up his mind and his closet. I can't picture a redneck wearing clogs, and they're probably not a big seller in Arlington, Texas.

I did learn that you have to go downstairs carefully in clogs. Not only are they a bit loose due to not having laces, but mine have a two-inch heel. One day, while wearing my clogs, I was walking to my car located behind the hospital. I would take a little shortcut through a small field of weeds to get to my car. As I walked towards the field, I noticed a Suburban SUV about to park in a compact space. My wife parks her large Toyota Highlander in compact spots too. Anyway, this Suburban caught my attention as there was a car to the right of this space. On the left side of the parking space was a curb, marking the end of the parking lot. I couldn't see how she was going to park in the small space.

The Suburban went up on the curb and came back down, landing the SUV perfectly back on the ground and into the space. I was so fascinated with this that I wasn't watching where I was walking. I tripped on the curb and found myself falling into the weeds. I thought that if my legs could catch up to my body, I could regain my balance and not fall. Thus, I started to run, but the next thing I knew, I felt as though I was sliding into third base headfirst.

As I was sliding through the dirt, I thought, "Oh my God, I don't care if I'm hurt. I just hope nobody is watching this." Unfortunately, the whole thing was seen by the hospital's purchasing manager John. He turned his head away to pretend he didn't see me so as not to embarrass me further.

I picked myself up and quickly walked to my car. I didn't even bother to brush myself off. I just got into my car and drove off. It was then that I realized I had dried weeds caught in my hair.

I was telling a friend of mine about my recent discovery of clogs. Dan and I did our OB/GYN residencies together many years ago in Los Angeles. He and I have quite different personalities, but somehow, as lowly residents, we became friends. It was as though we had become cellmates in prison. We hung out with our fellow residents during our residency, as we thought there was strength in numbers against a common enemy. Our enemy was our residency, which was the last hurdle between us and our ultimate goal of becoming practicing physicians. Today he practices in Orange County, California. On hearing of my enthusiasm for clogs, he confessed to me the following story that I found difficult to believe.

He said, "Gary, I've never mentioned this to anyone, but I not only share your enthusiasm for clogs, but I also have a clog fetish. I once took the bus from Newport Beach to the City of Orange and saw a woman at the back of the bus wearing beautiful red patent leather clogs. I couldn't resist sitting next to her, introducing myself, and complimenting her on her beautiful clogs. I was very excited, and before I could stop myself, I asked her if I could suck on her toes. To my surprise, she 'whipped them out.' We were in the back of an empty bus, so no one saw us."

I must have looked very surprised because Dan asked, "Why do you look so shocked?"

I replied, "Whoa, whoa, whoa. That story is unbelievable."

Dan asked, "What is unbelievable about it?"

I replied, "I can't believe you are a doctor, and you take the bus."

Chapter 11

Code Stork

At our hospital, we have some codes that are announced over the loudspeaker to alert us to specific emergencies. These codes are somewhat universal in that they are used in all hospitals to some extent. Everyone has heard the term "code blue." It means that a patient is turning blue from either a cardiac and/or a pulmonary arrest.

One of the codes that we used to use was called "code stork." When I first heard it, I thought they were saying "code dork," and I thought it meant there was an immediate need for a hospital administrator. Code stork signified an impending baby's delivery but with no physician around to deliver it. It was like saying, "Is there a doctor in the house?"

One day an overhead page went out at our hospital: "Any obstetrician to labor and delivery, stat! Any obstetrician to labor and delivery, stat!" One minute later, a new announcement went out: "Any doctor to labor and delivery, stat! Any doctor to labor and delivery, stat!"

An anesthesiologist, Dr. James, and a spine surgeon, Dr. Santi, were waiting for their next surgical case in the doctor's lounge. They had heard the first call and just ignored it. After hearing the second call, they ran up the stairs to the labor and delivery suite on the second floor. They arrived short of breath. A nurse ran out of a patient's room and shouted to the two doctors, "The heart rate is down to 60!" The surgeon looked at the anesthesiologist and asked, "Is that the mother's or the baby's heart rate? Dr. James responded, "It's the baby's." Dr. Santi then asked, "Is that good or bad?" Dr. James replied, "That's bad."

As doctors become more expert and experienced in their chosen specialty, the less expert and comfortable they become with the other specialties.

Chapter 12

A Doctor Named Phuc

The pregnant woman I had just admitted was 34 weeks pregnant. She had a fever, was short of breath, and had an abnormal chest X-ray. The fetal heart rate was rapid, but otherwise normal. I had to get an internal medicine consult to manage her pneumonia, as I was not an expert at managing non-pregnancy illnesses.

It turned out that the internal medicine doctor available that day was Vietnamese, and his name was Phuc Nguyen. He quickly came down from the Intensive Care Unit (I.C.U.) to help me.

The following conversation took place between us.

Me: Doctor, how do you pronounce your name?"

Phuc: Well, my first name is pronounced similar to how it is spelled, and my last name is pronounced: "Win."

Me: Hmm, I'm sure you are aware that there is an English word that sounds very similar to your first name.

Phuc: (laughing): I am very much aware of that.

Me: I wish that were my first name. If that were my first name, I would change my last name to Yoon.

Phuc: (laughing harder): Can you imagine?

Me: I can imagine a highway patrolman stopping me and saying, "What is your name, son?" I would respond, "Phuc Yoon."

"Hey, don't get smart with me," he would respond.

Me: Have you ever thought of changing your name to say, Phillip? I like that name.

Phuc: Do I look like a Phillip? That name is too Anglo-sounding. A familiar name in my country is Ho, but a woman with that name would not come to this country and change it to Penelope.

Me: I see your point.

Phuc: Some Vietnamese men with my first name change their name to Frank when they come here, but I decided to keep the name my parents gave me. Would you change your name to Dang just because you moved to Viet Nam? Would you want to lose your American identity?

Me: Again, you make a good point. I would consider taking the name Dong, but you are right; I would probably leave my name the same. I like the American name my parents gave me even though my ancestors are from Japan.

Me: My mother's first name was Fumi. She grew up in San Francisco and wanted an American name, so she went by Lilly. A lot of Asian Americans, including Chinese women, go by that name.

Me: Is it okay to call you by your first name? You can call me Gary.

Phuc: Yes, of course. You may find this amusing. I know a woman whose name is Bich, which means jade. It is not pronounced the same as the English word "bitch," but if someone were reading it phonetically, they would pronounce it "bitch"' I think she should change her name.

Me: You know what, Phuc? She should definitely change her name. That's embarrassing.

Phuc: What name would you suggest?

Me: I think Bianca is a pretty name and the two first letters of the names are the same.

Phuc: That is an excellent recommendation. I will suggest that to her. When my sister came to the U.S., she had people call her Kim, a Vietnamese and an American name.

Me: Ah, that is what we would call a "win-win." Do you get it? That is a win, Nguyen.

Phuc: Yes, I get it. That is a play on my last name.

Later, I was sitting down and placing orders on the computer. Phuc was standing at the nurse's station, studying the patient's obstetrical records. I called out from across the room.

Me: Phuc, do you think we should order blood cultures?

Suddenly, all the nurses at the nurse's station looked my way.

Phuc: That is a good idea. Do you want me to put in the orders?

Me: Phuc, yes. That would be a big help.

Phuc: Gary, you didn't want her placed in the I.C.U., did you?

Me: Phuc, no. I thought we would keep her here in the O.B. unit unless she gets worse. The nurses up there get very nervous if they have to take care of a pregnant woman. Their greatest fear is that the woman will go into labor while in their unit.

Phuc: Gary, which one of us is going to be the admitting doctor?

Me: Phuc, me. I am the admitting doc. You are the consultant.

I was having too much fun calling out Phuc's name, but now he was on to me. He smiled. I had just made a new friend.

I felt that I had accomplished something. In a small way, I was promoting diplomacy. If a Japanese and a Vietnamese can make fun of themselves (mostly me making fun of him) and laugh, maybe there is hope for all of us.

As Phuc was leaving, he noted, "Gary, this is the third pregnant woman I have consulted on this week and I had not seen a pregnant woman for months. What do we call it when we see an unexpectedly large number of cases?"

I responded, "I think we call it a cluster, Phuc."

Chapter 13

Massage Therapy as a Treatment for Stress

I believe that the stress of my job was killing me, literally. I have never smoked yet I developed lung cancer. Some would say that I developed lung cancer because surgeons breathe in some of the smoke that is emitted from the cautery that is used to stop bleeding in surgery. However, I am not aware that surgeons have a higher incidence of lung cancer than the general public. No, I believe I developed lung cancer because of stress. Of course, I cannot prove it.

According to biographer Walter Isaacson, Steve Jobs believed that his pancreatic cancer resulted from an extremely stressful time in his life when he led Apple and Pixar in the late 1990s. One must add, however, although Jobs was a genius, he was not very smart when it came to his own healthcare decisions. He chose not to receive treatment that may have saved his life.

In my personal case, I find my stress comes from having a heavy workload. This workload for me is largely because of trying to keep up with the electronic medical records, significant deliveries, and E.R. visits in the middle of the night. This leads to exhaustion, reduced job satisfaction, and physical illness.

There was a study done in 2015 on intensive care nurses at the Isfahan University of Medical Sciences in Iran. 66 male and female nurses were randomly divided into two groups. One group received massage therapy, and the other was a control group. The questionnaires were given before, immediately after the intervention, and two weeks after the completion of the study. The experimental group received Swedish massage therapy for four weeks, two times a week for 25 minutes. The Occupational Stress Inventory (OSI) was completed by the participants before and after the intervention.

Direct medical costs associated with stress-related problems in the United States are estimated to be about 300 billion dollars. One study showed that 7% of nurses are absent per week due to disability caused by stress, which is 80% higher than in other professions. It is known that high levels of occupational stress cause an increase in physical illness.

One of the non-pharmaceutical methods of reducing stress is massage therapy. Massage therapy has beneficial physiological effects such as improvement in the lymphatic and venous circulation, mental well-being, and stress reduction. It has also been found to decrease sleep disturbance, decrease blood pressure, and heart rate.

What were the results of the above-mentioned study? The control group received no benefit. The massage group's occupational stress was significantly lower immediately after the intervention. I was surprised to see that the stress remained low in the experimental group two weeks after the massage therapy had ended!

It would be nice if we could get rid of the stressors in our lives, but that is not always possible. I am a strong believer in massage as a way to combat stress and the toll it takes on society and us individually.

Chapter 14

Asian Massage Parlor

One day the nurses and receptionists in our obstetrical unit asked me if I would like to join them on a Friday trip to an Indian casino called Cache Creek Casino Resort. They told me the day trip would consist of eating and swimming, but the highlight was that everyone would be getting a one-hour massage. I told them I would love to join them, but I had never received a professional massage. They told me I was about to discover one of life's greatest rewards.

When we arrived at the resort, I realized that out of seven of us making the trip, I was the only male. I didn't know whether to be flattered or insulted. Many questions went through my mind. Was I considered "one of the girls?" Were they comfortable being in their swimsuits with me because I did not have an impressive physique? I decided to just enjoy the day. I thought, whatever the reason, they must be comfortable having me around and I enjoyed being with them.

When we got into the swimming pool with our drinks, I asked, "Can you feel the water getting warmer?" They responded with "No." I said, "How about now?" They looked at each other and then broke out laughing.

It turned out the massage was a wonderful experience. I knew that I had become addicted and would spend years seeking out the best massage therapists just as wine aficionados seek out the best wines.

I shared my massage experience with my haircutter. She worked at a place called Electric Beach. It was called that because it was also a tanning salon. My wife once got a spray tan there. I asked her why she did that. She said, "If you are tanned, you don't look fat. You look fit." I said, "Really, have you ever seen the movie *Big Momma's House*?"

Once while there, I saw one of my pregnant patients going in to get a tan in one of their tanning beds. She said to me, "I'm so glad you're here because I want to ask you if it is safe for me to tan while I am pregnant." I told her it was safe for the baby, but not so safe for her own skin. She said, "That is not a problem, as I always wear sunscreen in the tanning bed." I replied, "Alrighty then, good times."

It turned out that my haircutter (she says she is my stylist), Laura, was very fond of getting massages, so we decided from that day forward, we would share stories of good and bad massage experiences. Laura told me she had gone to a superb massage therapist, but the therapist wouldn't stop talking. I told her that I had the solution to that problem. I recommended that she make small talk for the first few minutes to be cordial, and then stop talking. Laura asked, "What do you do if she still keeps talking?" I told her to say, "Save it, bitch." I wouldn't really say that. Massage therapists will get the message if you make your answers to their questions very short. As a last resort, you can start snoring. I have at times caught myself snoring even though I do my best to stay awake. I don't want to wake up to find that the massage is over. When I snore, it is usually just a single snort, and that wakes me up. I then end up laughing, as does the therapist.

Laura told me about a new massage spa that she had just discovered called Paradiso Health Spa. It was located near Electric Beach. She said she generally would not have gone there as it looked a bit shady, but a client had recommended the place, and the prices were very reasonable. I thought it would make more sense to get a massage in a hair salon or a chiropractic/health center because that way one knows that the massage therapist is part of a legitimate place of business. The massage salon Laura was recommending only offered massage.

I decided to drive into the strip mall's parking lot where the massage studio was located just to see if it looked safe. I noticed an American flag and a Liberty Bell sign at a place called By The People. It looked like a do-it-yourself legal assistance store that could help you fill out simple documents without a lawyer. I imagined they could help you manage a friendly divorce or change the legal name of your dog.

Next, there was a Mongolian tailor shop, a karate studio, and a nail salon. There was also a place called Tasty Indian Pizza restaurant. I like Indian food, and I like pizza, so why not? I have been told that they have the best Indian pizza in town.

There is also a Chinese takeout restaurant there. My Chinese friend Richard eats there. He gives it a mixed review. He likes the fact that there are no crowds, and the portions are generous with noodles overflowing from their Styrofoam takeout boxes. His only complaint is that he doesn't care for their food.

With so many nationalities represented, the strip mall looked like a ghetto Epcot Center. Overall, I thought the strip mall looked safe enough.

I decided to continue my vetting process by checking online reviews to make certain this was a legitimate place of business. I found 81 reviews from a nationally recognized website that I usually use for restaurant recommendations.

Many of the reviews gave the highest rating of five stars. I didn't really need to read those. I wanted to read the one-star reviews to see if there were any red flags. One woman, Darlene P., wrote, "I have been going to this place for years. I found a male therapist that was very good. I asked for him exclusively each time. I'd say I've had at least ten massages from him that were consistently good. The last time I went, he was grinding against me with his hips and he had an erection. I was so very shocked, I couldn't move. I should have left without paying, but because he took seventy minutes and it was a rather good massage, besides the grinding, I felt it was the right thing to pay. I couldn't communicate because his English wasn't good, so I left feeling violated. I'll never go back. I gave him a 20% tip."

The website showed a thumbnail picture of the Asian woman owner. The following is her verbatim response. "The masseur you said has been fired. We only do massage and nothing else. We want our customer to come happy and go home satisfied."

The wording of that last sentence was unfortunate but the owner's communication skills are not bad considering English is her second language. I was surprised to see that she knew the word "masseur." Under the circumstances, the tip and the two stars given by the customer seemed overly generous.

The manager finished with, "I hope see you again."

There was another review that was similar by Bella D. If I understand her correctly, her massage therapist rested his penis on her back while she was receiving her massage. At first, she couldn't believe it was happening. She then tried to convince herself that this was a cultural thing.

Massage therapists are taught to try to have physical contact with the client until the massage has ended. I have had massage therapists drag one hand on my back as they went from one side of my body to the other. The constant contact is calming, the flow is not interrupted, and you know where the therapist is at all times so you won't be startled. Some therapists use a holster to carry their oil, so they never have to leave the client and reach for their oil. Maybe the therapist thought he had invented some bizarre hands free way of letting the client know where he was at all times. The client said that she would not be returning to this establishment.

There was one last horrendous review. Calvina H. wrote, "The shoddy tables squeak and make noise. So about fifteen minutes into my ninety-minute massage, I heard a noise, but I chose to assume it was the table.

Unfortunately, I was wrong. The massage therapist had just farted. And it was no benign fart. It was FULLY LOADED and about knocked me out when I smelled it."

I thought, "Fully Loaded? Who talks like that?"

Calvina continued, "I held my breath, it was so bad. I felt bad for the lady, though, and figured she was probably pretty embarrassed. I stopped feeling bad for her when she farted again… and again… at LEAST six times during my ninety-minute massage. In that tiny room… basically hotboxing."

I had never heard of hotboxing, so I looked it up. Apparently, people will find a small enclosed non-ventilated space to smoke marijuana (or hashish) to intensify the effect of the smoke.

Calvina went on, "Look, I get that digestive issues happen and it sucks. But if you are having crazy gas and you're a massage therapist, excuse yourself and let someone else take over for you!"

I wish I knew Calvina. She has colorful language and apparently leads an interesting life.

There are at least two massage salons near my hometown that are not legitimate. One is near the police station. They get shut down occasionally, but then they open right back up again. When they were raided, they would fine the owner and print the names of the clients in the local newspaper. One of the prominent lawyers in town got busted. His name was published in the paper, so he called all his clients to apologize and encourage them to continue doing business with him. The clients told him that they didn't read the small-town newspaper and would have never known he had been busted. Besides, no one assumed that he was a man of high moral character, as they already knew he was a lawyer.

The things that distinguish these two massage places from legitimate establishments are the following: They are both run totally by Asians, they are open until 10 pm when all other downtown businesses are closed, and most of their customers do not make an appointment. The customers without an appointment are called "walk-ins." An acronym for this type of establishment is A.M.P., which stands for Asian Massage Parlor.

Based on this information, you can imagine my trepidation when I walked into the massage spa and saw that only Asian women were present, it was open late, and they could take me immediately. As I had driven up to the establishment, I noticed that the massage spa had a small red neon sign that flashed, "MASSAGE."

On the other hand, I knew Laura would not give me bad advice, and I was looking forward to their low prices.

My massage therapist was to be Amy. The other choices were Jennifer, CI-Ci, and Cynthia. I thought these were curious names, considering these women did not speak English. Only the receptionist spoke English. I asked Amy where she was from. She said she was from China. I asked her if Amy was a common name in China. She giggled. I told her I thought her real name should be "You Pay Now." She giggled again, but she couldn't understand what I was saying. She was just being polite.

She showed me to my room and left while I undressed. I noticed there was a washcloth folded neatly on a small table in the dimly lit room. It looked a bit stiff and scratchy, but it also appeared clean. I thought, "Why would we need a washcloth?" There was also a bottle of oil and a box of tissues on the table.

I stripped down to just my underwear and laid down prone on the massage table. Amy came in and saw that I had my underwear on. She just stood there and looked at me as though I was wearing a three-piece suit. She then, without saying a word, jerked my underwear down to my knees. I then said, "Whoa, whoa, whoa," but without saying a word, she started massaging. Apparently, "Whoa, whoa, whoa," in Chinese means, "Thank you for taking off my underwear." Amy spoke very little English, or she would have explained that one cannot get a good massage of the buttocks muscles with underwear on. She knew that your buttocks muscles are one of the largest muscle groups in the body.

To have a massage of the buttocks with underwear on would be as awkward as performing a Pap smear with the patient's underwear still on. It could be done, but not easily. I once had a Hispanic patient that couldn't understand that she had to get undressed for her gynecologic exam. I entered the exam room only to find her fully clothed. In my broken Spanish, I said, "Usted, no necesita pantalones (pants), por favor." When I returned in a few minutes, she was still fully dressed. I finally went through the pantomime motions of stepping out of my pants and then pretended to squirm out of my underwear. I then mimicked the motions of shooting the underwear to the chair using the elastic band. A big smile of recognition came over her face.

The following week I returned to get another massage from Amy. This time, after I undressed, I pulled my underwear down to my knees and then took my place on the table. I then placed the sheet over myself. When Amy entered the room and realized what I had done with my underwear, she just stood there without saying a word. She then jerked them totally off of me and tossed my underwear onto my stack of clothing. Again, I said, "Whoa, whoa, whoa," but again, she just went on with the massage. Since then, I decided I would never wear underwear again during a massage. It takes a bit to get used to having that much exposure, but eventually you feel that it is all clinical, no different than if you were in the doctor's office receiving an exam.

Most of the female nurses that I have discussed this with do not wear underwear while receiving a massage, but men have a problem that women don't have. Men flop around a bit. At some point, the massage therapist will have you turn over onto your back. All the massage therapists I have ever been to are very discreet. They take the sheet that is covering you and hold it up while you turn over. The problem is what position your "male member" will take now that you are on your back. I turned over and hoped that he would fall into the standard anatomic and most acceptable 6 o'clock position. This was never an issue when I was wearing my "tighty whities." When I had underwear on, I knew he would stay put because of the underwear support. Now, with "the flop," anything goes.

Fortunately for me, when I did my flip from prone to supine, I fell into the 6:00 position. I almost stood up and cheered, but that would have been awkward. It was as though I had achieved a "perfect dismount." If this were an Olympic event, I might have received a 10. I pictured Jennifer, Ci-Ci, and Cynthia walking into our room with signs that read: 9.9, 9.8, and 9.9. Unfortunately, my victory was short-lived. As I centered myself on the table, my "appendage" moved to the 4:30 position. Oh no, then he slipped to 4:00. If he moves to 3:00, one of us is going to have to move him! It is not as though I am hanging off the table's edge, but it is still embarrassing. I thought, "Maybe it is only embarrassing for me."

As the massage continued, I resumed enjoying my massage. Then suddenly, I got the feeling that I might be sticking out of the sheet on my left. I thought that I might have moved to 3:00. I thought, "No, if that were the case, she would have seen him in the dim light and have given him a little nudge to get him back under the sheet. At that moment, she was working on my right leg. When it came time to work on my left leg, she looked and saw that I was a bit exposed. She did not know how to say "sorry" in English, so she said, "Oh, soddy." She then reached behind her for that white washcloth that was on her small table. The washcloth was there for moments like this.

Do you know how you might pick up dog poop in your backyard with a paper towel? Well, she picked me up with the washcloth and carefully placed me back under the sheet. She then put down the washcloth. I almost started laughing but thought I had best not make a scene. She might think I was being inappropriate and have me kicked out.

I later told my O.B. partner, Amy, about my experience. She is from Israel, very discriminating and blunt. As an expert on all types of massage, I looked forward to her advice. She said, "Gary, you should never wear your underwear when you are getting a massage. Do you think you have something that people are dying to see? Well, you don't!"

Chapter 15

Oxycodone and Me

I pretty much have no vices. I have no interest in alcohol, tobacco, marijuana, gambling, etc. In this respect, I am rather boring.

Despite that, I feel that I am just one bad decision away from becoming an opioid addict. I have had a number of surgeries over the last few years. After the surgery, I usually take opioids for a few days.

The feeling that I get from opioids is one of peace. I can best describe this feeling by citing quotes from others. Author Maya Angelou described a lavender Easter dress that she was going to wear as a child. She fantasized that the dress had magical powers and she "… was going to look like one of the sweet little white girls who was everybody's dream of what was right with the world." I feel all is right with the world when on opioids.

Another quote comes from comedian Lenny Bruce who was addicted to heroin and morphine. He was aware of the pleasures and perils of taking opioids. The following quote is attributed to him: "I'll die young, but it's like kissing God." He died from an overdose at age 40.

Opioids are the only thing that I have found that can give me a complete break from the angst of daily life. Nothing else can compare. For example, I do not find sleep to be very refreshing as I often have dreams that are anxiety provoking such as dreaming that I am about to take an exam I am unprepared for.

Recently, I had heart surgery. On the day after surgery, I was to be discharged home. The nurse practitioner asked me if I would like any meds to take at home. I said, "Yes, I would like oxycodone 5 mg. every 4-6 hours. Please dispense 5 tablets total. I will not call for refills, as I will take plain Tylenol if I continue to have pain." Normally, healthcare providers do not like being told by the patient exactly what prescription they want, including the dosage. This is particularly true when it comes to narcotics, as it is a clue that the patient is seeking addictive drugs. The nurse practitioner knew that I was a doctor and since I asked for such a small number of pills, she just smiled and sent the prescription to my pharmacy electronically.

On the way home, I stopped at my pharmacy and waited my turn to pick up my prescription. The pharmacy tech, Betsy, and I have been on friendly terms since the first day that I came to her counter. On that first day, she recognized me as her mother's doctor, though I am now retired.

At this visit, Betsy said, "Hi Dr. Matsumura, we have your prescription ready. Here is your oxycodone and naloxone." I said, "Wait a minute Betsy, my doctor did not order any naloxone." (Naloxone is used to reverse the effects of an opioid in the event of an overdose. For example, overdosing can cause one to be unresponsive or even stop breathing, but those effects can be reversed.) Betsy said, "Well, doctors now routinely prescribe naloxone with narcotics in case you overdose." I said, "I am not going to overdose on my five pills." Betsy replied, "No, not that kind of overdose. It is in case you try to commit suicide."

I looked behind me to see if anyone was waiting in line to pick up their prescription. Fortunately, there was not, so I continued, "Whoa, what makes you think I am going to commit suicide? I can tell you, Betsy, I have no such plans, but if I were going to commit suicide, it might be because I was suffering from terminal cancer. If that were the case, I would not want the antidote."

Betsy smiled and then said, "Well, there is an opioid epidemic in this country. What if you come across someone who has overdosed on opioids? You could save their life."

Betsy said, "You know, I am just the messenger. I did not write the prescription. I am just a lowly pharmacy tech."

I said, "Betsy, don't you sell yourself short. I delivered you and you turned out to be an intelligent trained professional. You must have had to take a weekend online course to get to where you are." I winked.

Betsy stepped back, pretending to be offended, but then laughed and said, "My mother always said you were funny. Now I understand what she meant."

The opioid epidemic began in the late 1990s. That was when the Sacklers' Purdue Pharma started aggressively marketing highly addictive opioids such as OxyContin.

Another wave of opioid overdosage began in 2013 with illicit fentanyl, a powerful synthetic opioid that has become an overwhelming problem.

It turns out that my home state of California and nine other states have laws that require prescribers to prescribe or at least offer a prescription for naloxone when prescribing a schedule II opioid. It turns out that almost every person who has died of a witnessed opioid overdose could have been saved if the person with them had naloxone on them. Naloxone is not available without a prescription and many individuals would not normally request a prescription, as there is a stigma in asking for it. Thus, there is an effort being made to get more naloxone out in the community.

From 1999 to 2019, nearly 500,000 died from an overdose of opioids, according to the CDC. For comparison, there were about 300,000 U.S. combat deaths in World War II.

I recently read the highly acclaimed book *Empire of Pain: The Secret History of the Sackler Dynasty* by Patrick Radden Keefe. The book made my blood boil. By aggressively promoting OxyContin, the Sackler family's Purdue Pharma was able to get doctors to routinely prescribe OxyContin for pain (originally for severe but later for even moderate pain). They were able to convince an F.D.A. director to say that it was less addicting than similar narcotics when it was in fact more addicting. The F.D.A. regulator later got a very high-paying position at Purdue Pharma. The Sackler family made billions of dollars.

The family patriarch, Arthur Sackler, had nothing to do with OxyContin and yet the first third of the 560-page book is about him. He was the marketing genius behind the first pharmaceutical blockbuster, the tranquilizer Valium. His heirs would become marketing experts of OxyContin.

As the oldest of four children in the 1960s, I remember asking my mother why she took Valium. She laughed and said, "It is because I had too many children." In the 1970s, it became the most prescribed drug in the U.S. The Rolling Stones called it "Mother's Little Helper" in their 1966 hit song.

Large numbers do not really portray human suffering the way individual stories do. I decided to watch the Hulu series *Dopesick* so I could feel the impact the opioid epidemic had on individuals. The movie series is based on the non-fiction book of the same name by Beth Macy and stars Michael Keaton. Keaton plays a doctor that is loosely based on an actual doctor that not only got patients addicted to OxyContin, but became addicted himself. When one of his young addicted patients dies (a patient that he had delivered as a newborn), the doctor has overwhelming guilt. I found that scene to be emotionally moving. I suddenly could feel empathy for the tortured, hopeless addicts. Keaton does not play a hero. At his best, he feels conflicted. At his worst, he feels hopeless.

I believe the opioid crisis has adversely affected how we deal with Covid. Many Americans now believe that if you cannot trust Big Pharma and the F.D.A., then why would you trust the C.D.C. or Dr. Fauci, when in fact, they have done their best to save lives with the information that they had at the time on the novel coronavirus.

Dr. Fauci did not initially think that the general public needed to wear masks. I would be more critical of Dr. Fauci myself, but all of us physicians have had to second-guess ourselves. We then take in new information and move forward. There is a reason we call it the *practice* of medicine.

I retired from practicing medicine a few years ago, so I asked my friend Ned Levine, a urologist, about the naloxone mandate. He told me that when he orders an opioid in the electronic record, it automatically adds a prescription for naloxone. He said, however, "One can check a box and that will cancel the order for naloxone. I have checked off that box." I asked him, "Why?" He said, "Once I had a patient that called me back and went on an annoying rant about how he didn't need the naloxone."

In *Dopesick*, the despair of the addicts is heart-wrenching. I think watching that series has prevented at least one person from being tempted to abuse opioids—me.

Chapter 16

Embarrassing Tattoos

Iknow a physician named Dr. Douglas who has a reputation for thinking he "knows it all." Dr. James told me that Dr. Douglas is a dermatologist. I responded, "I thought Dr. Douglas was a family doctor." "No," said Dr. James, "he's a dermatologist because he thinks he knows the skin and all its contents."

Physicians see a lot of skin and thus also end up seeing a lot of tattoos. I try not to mention things like piercings of the genitals, tan lines, and tattoos when I examine patients. It wouldn't be very professional.

Sometimes a tattoo jumps out at you, and it can be challenging to ignore it. Other times, a tattoo is so "out there" that the patient mentions it, rather than waiting for you to say something.

I once saw a woman who had shaved off her pubic hair and on her mons pubis, she had a tattoo in large block letters. It looked like a homemade job. The tattoo read: ROBERT'S CANDY. At first, I didn't know what that meant. Then I realized it referred to her genital area. I must have looked startled because the patient said to me, "What do you think of my tattoo?"

I didn't know what to say. I said, "Uh… well, what do you think of it?" This is a good technique. When you are uncomfortable with a question, answer it with another question. It takes you off the hot seat and gives you more time to formulate an answer.

She replied, "Well, it's a problem." I asked, "What do you mean?"

She said, "Well, Robert is no longer in the picture. What do you think I should do?"

"Well," I replied, "You could sign up with a computer dating service and tell them you are only interested in men named Robert. Then the first time your new Robert sees it he will be very impressed with your early commitment. You could seek professional help to try to remove the tattoo. One option would be to have the skin excised like a mini tummy tuck, but that would be painful, and insurance won't cover it. I imagine the tattoo could be turned into some other design."

She responded, "I like the tattoo. I just wish Robert's name wasn't there."

I then said, "You should have had the tattoo say, YOUR NAME HERE." She laughed.

I know a colleague who had a negative experience with a patient and her tattoo. The woman was what we call a "walk-in," that is, she came into our hospital in labor but didn't have a doctor, so she was assigned to the doctor on call for unassigned patients.

When she lifted her gown, a large tattoo on her lower white abdomen read, in block letters: "TRUST NO NIGGERS." Her attending physician that night was Dr. Washington. He is a black obstetrician. Dr. Washington was very professional. He didn't ask for a different physician to take his place. He just took care of the patient. The patient explained: "The tattoo doesn't mean what you think." Dr. Washington didn't pursue it further. I would have asked, "Oh, well then, what does it mean? Maybe you could use it in a sentence." I wouldn't have put her on the spot like that. I feel sorry for her. She must regret getting that tattoo.

The "N-word" is so offensive and derogatory that I was reluctant to even bring it up in this context. My daughter wanted to read *Adventures of Huckleberry Finn*. She did not want the "N-word" to get stuck in her head, so she used an e-book manager to convert that word to "negro" before the book was uploaded to her e-reader.

The patient named her baby Roy. Ironically, that was Dr. Washington's first name. I don't know if she knew that was his first name. Then again, maybe she did know and was looking for redemption.

Chapter 17

Italian Job

My perfect dream job would be to work in Italy. I live in Fairfield, California. It is a military town as Travis Air Force Base is located there. Many of the physicians in the community are Air Force veterans, as was my OB/GYN partner of twenty-five years. Some of my colleagues were able to retire from the military with full retirement benefits and then work as civilian physicians.

I often envied these men and women who served their countries and now have lifelong friends throughout the U.S. as well as in countries such as Germany and Japan. I assumed that when I retired, almost all of my friends would be from my hometown, where I have lived most of my life. I often wondered if I was missing out.

When I first moved to Fairfield, I joined a multispecialty medical group. One of the senior physicians there was very well respected. His first name was Ron. For the next forty years, he would call me Gary, but I never felt comfortable calling him by his first name. I always respectfully called him Dr. Nakamura.

He had been a colonel in the Air Force and was working at the group that I had joined. He tried to take me under his wing as he had been the director of a residency program and I had just completed my residency. I also think he wanted to mentor me because we were both of Japanese ancestry. I did not want to be mentored, as I had a bit of an independent streak. I was tired of the residency hierarchy where every attending physician and professor was able to boss or even intimidate the residents.

Somehow, Dr. Nakamura found out I had protested the Vietnam War while I was in high school. He said to me, "While you were protesting the war, I was in Vietnam serving my country." I replied, "If we had not protested, you might still be there."

I regret today that I responded in such an arrogant manner. I would be much more modest today, but I must have been a haughty thirty-year-old doctor at the time, out to prove myself. As time would go on, there was a lot that I would learn from experienced doctors like Dr. Nakamura. It turns out that residency is not the end of one's training; it is the beginning. Even in my last year of practice, I took courses to improve my surgical skills and deal with obstetrical emergencies.

Despite my haughty response to Dr. Nakamura, he and I became friends. I enjoyed the stories of his travels throughout the world and of his time in the military. He told me that during the Vietnam War he would be operating long hours in the hospital when a patient would arrive on his floor by elevator. The patient had been sent by elevator from the maternity ward. There would be a note pinned to her gown that only said, "Needs C-section." His surgical team would do the cesarean and send the patient back down the elevator with the baby and no note.

Near the end of my career, I had become experienced enough that OB/GYN physicians would sometimes ask for my help in difficult cases such as delivering the second twin in a vaginal delivery or dealing with uncontrolled bleeding during a cesarean section.

I was able to get to know the OB/GYN physicians from David Grant Medical Center (DGMC) which was the hospital at Travis Air Force Base. These physicians would transfer high-risk obstetrical patients to our hospital since we had a neonatal intensive care unit, and they did not. I was impressed with these young physicians. They were very knowledgeable and competent even though they were very young. I loved to see them come to our hospital in their camouflage uniforms and boots. I don't feel disdain for the military as I did in high school when I protested the Vietnam War. These men and women in the armed services are willing to put themselves in harm's way for my family and me. I make a point of thanking them for their service.

I got to know a few of them well enough to recognize their voices on the phone. I was disappointed to find that almost all of these active-duty physicians would move on after a couple of years.

I wondered if I taught in a teaching program, would I be one of those doctors that was condescending to residents? I don't believe I would be, but maybe after many years of practicing medicine, residents and young doctors may appear to only have an elementary knowledge of the specialty. I do remember losing my patience with a doctor at DGMC that was trying to transfer a patient to me. I think the patient had twins and was soon to deliver at thirty-seven weeks' gestation. I did not see why this patient needed to be transferred to our hospital, even though we could offer a higher level of care. After arguing a bit, I relented, as the transferring physician was just following her department's protocols.

Near the end of my career, I had a fantasy that possibly I could travel the world and help young doctors in the military. I found that there was a U.S. Naval Hospital in Naples, Italy. I thought this would be perfect. I called a Navy Recruitment Center and told them I wanted to join the Navy and be stationed in Naples. I learned that I was too old to join the Navy and that recruits could not be guaranteed that they would be assigned to Naples.

Well, it was just a pipe dream. I should probably have visited Italy before making a life-changing decision, anyway. If I really loved Italy and wanted to live there, I could still probably find a way to do contract work in Naples as a civilian doctor. I booked a trip to Italy for my wife and me.

Our tour started in Rome. Having never been there before, we were very excited. Our group tour guide told us that eighty-five percent of the world's antiquities resided in Italy. I don't know if that is true and I am not going to look it up because I want it to be true, whether it is or not.

Our Italian tour company provided us with a "free" welcome dinner. We were very excited to try antipasti and pizza from the people who invented those dishes. On the way to the restaurant, one of the American tourists remarked that there were many pizzerias in Italy. He asked if they had been imported from America. We Americans are a very ethnocentric group.

We would have pizza many times during our stay in Italy. Although some of it was very good, overall, we found the pizza to be rather dry. We tried to get a *Maui Zowie* but found it is blasphemy to ask for pineapple on your pizza in Italy. They look at you as though you had asked for a shrimp gelato. We found that the spaghetti is also served on the dry side, without a lot of sauce. The Parmesan cheese, however, is robust, aged, and tasty. It is even better than the white dust that comes out of that tall green canister in the U.S.

Anyway, getting back to the first supper… People tend to drink a lot when they are on vacation, especially if the wine is complimentary and there is a designated motor coach driver to take them back to their hotel. As the dinner progressed, two musicians joined us. One played the flute. The other played the guitar and serenaded us. By then, each table had put away several bottles of wine.

The musicians would ask for volunteers to sing with them, and soon we had turned the restaurant into a karaoke bar. One of the women was feeling courageous from the wine and asked if she could sing "Volare." "Naturalmente," said the guitarist. Unfortunately, the only words she knew of the song were "Volare, oh oh, E cantare, oh oh oh oh," and that was it. She did manage to come in at the right times.

Not to be outdone, another woman asked if she could sing "Amore." The only words to the song that she knew were the beginning: "When the moon in the sky looks like a biga pizza pie, that's amore." The musicians knew many non-Italian popular songs that were remotely connected to Italians. They played the love theme from *Romeo and Juliet*, the Titanic movie theme: "My Heart Will Go On" (Leonardo Di Caprio), "Eye of the Tiger" (Sylvester Stallone), and "My Way" (Frank Sinatra).

One man in the group—actually it was me—asked the musicians if they could play "Moon River." They said they could, but one of my Aussie mates in the travel group didn't think "Moon River" had any connection to Italy. I said, "Of course it does. First of all, Henry Mancini wrote it, and second, it was performed by Andy Williams, who was married to Claudine Longet, who was French."

My new tablemate said, "But being French is not the same as being Italian."

"Well," I replied, "An Italian is basically a French person who is polite, capisce?" All right, he bought it, so I crooned, "Moon River, wider than a mile, I'm crossing you in style, somedaaay." The group loved it, not because of my singing, but because this mostly retired group of American tourists thinks of Andy Williams as a god.

I never did pursue practicing medicine in Italy. I soon found out that I had a life-threatening cancer and would need surgery followed by months of chemotherapy, but that was the furthest thing from my mind that night.

After dinner, the musicians came out again and asked if there were any other Italian favorites that they could play. A woman called out, "Country Roads by John

Denver." By this point, no one questioned if that was an Italian song. Apparently, we weren't the first group of inebriated Americans to request that classic song. Without missing a beat, the musicians started playing as we sang out: "Country roads, take me home, to the place, I be-loooong …." I sang along even though I don't really care for John Denver. I thought, when in Rome….

Chapter 18

Locum Tenens

Our practice had a good reputation, and our town was growing, so we found ourselves overwhelmed with patients. It was time for us to recruit a new obstetrician. By the time you advertise for a new obstetrician, do interviews, and wait for a physician to become available, it can take a year before you find someone to join you.

That's when you call a locum tenens company, and they will send you a "rent-a-doc." The locum tenens company is a physician temp service. Being naïve, I figured that these *locum tenens* doctors liked to travel and make new friends while still earning an income. They shouldn't need much screening. I was wrong. I suspect some of these physicians would have difficulty keeping a job in the real world, although I must say there are some excellent *locum tenens* physicians out there.

The first locum that I hired was Dr. Johnson. He was very personable. He was calm and reasonable. He was very active in volunteer work. I liked him immediately, and I was very proud of myself for finding and hiring him. I assumed that I was an excellent judge of character. He had worked with some of the well-known obstetricians in Northern California.

One day our nurse manager, Pauline, said to me, "We need to talk." That is never a good thing. "The doctor that you hired has a strange way of greeting women. He shakes their breast instead of their hand."

I said, "What?" Pauline replied, "You heard me. He shakes their breast instead of their hand."

"Whoa, whoa, whoa," I said. "His hand must have slipped or something."

"Well, he did it to two of our nurses now and one of the events was witnessed."

"Do you think these two nurses have a conspiracy against this doctor? Do they dislike him for some reason?" I asked.

"No, I don't think so. They both like him, and neither of them is complaining about it. They think that it's unusual. They didn't want to tell you about it for fear that you would fire him."

"Oh my God! I've got to tell our physician President, Dr. Levine."

I explained the situation to Dr. Levine, who immediately stood up and said, "We've got to fire this guy. We cannot tolerate such behavior!"

"I know, I know, but…but…." I was trying to find an excuse to give him a second chance. I really liked this doctor.

"But what?" said Dr. Levine.

"Well…" I was grasping at anything. "Well, what if in his culture that is how they greet women?"

"Okay, I had not thought of that. Where is he from?" asked Dr. Levine.

"Oakland," I replied. We fired him the next morning.

Chapter 19

Gender Issues

In an OB/GYN practice, on occasion, one deals with confusing gender orientation issues.

One day I was playing tennis with my urologist friend, Dr. Levine, when I received a call from the Emergency Room (E.R.). The E.R. doctor told me he needed me to attend to a sixteen-year-old lesbian girl bleeding from the vagina. The doctor then gave me a brief history of the patient over the phone. This girl was having sex with her female partner with a strap-on device and started bleeding rather briskly. Rather than coming immediately to the E.R., the patient waited until she had lost so much blood that she was dizzy. At that point, she asked her mother to take her to the hospital.

Dr. Levine overheard the word "strap-on" and wanted to know what was happening. I told him that I would have to cut our game short and go to the E.R. to take care of a patient. He asked, "If she has a bladder laceration are you going to ask me to come in and help you?" I responded, "Yes." "Well then," he replied, "you may as well tell me about her."

I explained the unusual case, and he got a puzzled look on his face. "If she wants a penis in her, why doesn't she have sex with a boy? The boy could wear a mask that made him look like a female."

I replied, "If she only likes females, she isn't going to want to have sex with a man. Nevertheless, there is satisfaction in filling the vagina. You wouldn't want to have sex with a man who was made up to look like a woman, would you?" I asked.

"No, no, I see your point," Dr. Levine quickly replied.

As I was driving to the E.R., I thought about my own life at that age. I was collecting baseball cards and Buffalo Head nickels. I hoped someday I could buy a Camaro or maybe even a '63 Corvette. I had found a discarded *Playboy* magazine at the apartment building where I did gardening. I knew I would want to see more of those magazines someday, but that could wait.

I was certainly not thinking about my sexuality at age sixteen. There would be plenty of time for that. The sixties were a slower time for a child. The *Super Mario Brothers* video game wouldn't be invented for decades. There was no *Sex and the City* for young people to watch. Lucy and Ricky Ricardo slept in separate beds wearing long-sleeved pajamas. I thought, "Kids nowadays don't take the time just to be kids." If I had added the word "shenanigans" in there somewhere, I would have sounded like my mother.

Fortunately, when I arrived at the E.R., I found that the patient's bleeding had almost stopped. I asked the girl why she had waited until she was dizzy before coming to the E.R. Now, she might need a blood transfusion.

"Well, what would you have done?" she asked. "Would you want to have to explain this situation to your mother?"

"No, you're right," I replied, "but I would have made something up."

"Like what?" she asked.

"Well, you could have said you were having a really heavy period, and you reached for a tampon but accidentally grabbed a letter opener."

I had intended to get her to relax a little, so I was pleased when she laughed.

"Seriously," I said, "you could have just said your period was out of control, and you needed to go to the hospital."

"Well," she replied, "I finally just told my mom the truth."

I responded, "That's really the best thing if you are comfortable with that."

The anesthesiologist read my history of the patient twice but was still puzzled. He was East Indian and was not familiar with some slang terms. After he had put the patient to sleep, he asked, "What is a strap-on device?"

"You've never heard of a strap-on device?" I asked.

"No," he replied.

"Well, you obviously don't watch enough H.B.O. You could learn a lot from this young girl." I explained that there were probably other names for this apparatus, but that was the term that I was familiar with. I then went on to explain to him what the device was.

He listened carefully and then exclaimed, "Ah yes, I am very familiar with this device." He did not elaborate.

Now that the patient was asleep, I could carefully assess the damage. I removed the packing that I had placed in the E.R. The bleeding had stopped. I found a two-centimeter tear at the top of the vagina. She would only need a few stitches. In a few minutes, her laceration was repaired.

The anesthesiologist remarked that he thought that lesbianism was perfectly normal. "If I were a woman," he stated, "I am certain that I would be a lesbian. I would not let some sweaty, hairy man get on top of me."

I countered with, "It's difficult for you to know if you would be a lesbian if you had been born a woman. You were born a man. Your brain is bathing in testosterone. Of course, you think you would like women under any circumstance."

He replied, "I often joke that I feel as though I'm a lesbian trapped in a man's body."

I then asked him, "Do you wish you were a woman?" He replied, "No, not at all." Then I said, "You have not thought this through very well. You are not a lesbian trapped in a man's body if you do not wish you were a woman. If you are trapped in a man's body that means you would prefer to be a woman."

He reluctantly agreed.

I went on: "I actually met a lesbian trapped in a man's body."

This particular woman was born a man but always felt that she was a woman, so she transitioned to a woman, yet she was only comfortable having sex with women. This had been true both before and after her sex change. She truly was "a lesbian trapped in a man's body."

"Hmm," said the anesthesiologist, "This is very confusing. I will have to think about that for a while." I responded, "I agree. It took me a while to get it all straight in my own head."

I had another patient that was even more confusing. It was confusing to me, but probably not to her. This patient was born a woman but wanted to be a man. She had both her uterus and ovaries removed. She used to take testosterone, so she grew a beard. She could no longer afford the testosterone, but the beard persisted. She only chose to have sex with men. This worked out well for her because she had a perfectly functioning vagina. This is where I have to concentrate, or I will confuse myself. This was a gay man trapped in a woman's body. Did I get that right?

The man having sex with her must feel he is a gay man having sex with a man who conveniently has a vagina.

Sexual identity can be very challenging. Some will undergo multiple surgeries. Others may want surgery but are hesitant. Family and friends alienate many of them. My heart goes out to these people who struggle, trying to decide whether to be true to their preferred sexuality or not.

Chapter 20

Answering Machine

I hate answering machines. I don't mind being put on hold as long as I can eventually talk to a human. Please let me talk to a human. How disingenuous is it to hear a recording that says, "Your call is very important to us."

Nevertheless, when I am not in the office, I have a voice machine that takes messages for me. Years ago, I tried to make my messages more interesting.

My first message said, "Hello, your message is very important to us. You have reached the phone of Dr. Matsumura. If you have a non-urgent medical question, you may call radio talk show host Dr. Dean Edell, or you may leave a message at the tone." One elderly woman left the following message: "Dr. Dean Edell…isn't he that guy on the radio? Why would I want to talk to him? Isn't he an eye doctor? That doesn't make any sense. I want to talk to my doctor. In the background, I could hear her friend yelling, 'Hang up! Hang up!'"

Too many people took that message seriously, so I deleted it.

My next message said, "Hello?" This was followed by a pause. Then I would again say, "Hello?" This was followed by a longer pause. Then I would say, "I'm not in now. Please leave a message."

Dr. Gary, an oncologist at U.C. Davis, responded to that message from his cell phone, "Hello, hello? Don't hang up. Can you hear me?" The next time he saw me, he said, "I think there's something wrong with your answering machine."

One day I was enjoying my lunch break while sitting at my office desk. I don't like to be interrupted while I'm taking my lunch break. I decided to answer the phone but pretend I was an answering machine so I wouldn't get caught up in a long conversation. The person calling was a family physician, Dr. Ottomon. He wanted to ask me a gynecologic question. I answered the phone with:

"Hello, welcome to Dr. Matsumura's proprietary *First Call Interactive* voice machine. Would you please state your name? Please speak slowly and clearly."

"Uh, my name is Dr. Ottomon."

"Now, if you speak English, press 1. If you speak Spanish, call Dr. Saavedra."

"Now, press 1 if you have an OB question, 2 if you have a GYN question, and 3 if you are looking for stock market recommendations."

After pressing 2, Dr. Ottomon said, "Well, I have been sending women to your nurse practitioner for Pap smears, but she doesn't always do them. For instance, if they have had a hysterectomy, she won't do them. Are Paps not indicated in those patients?"

"What are Pap smears for?" I asked.

The response was, "Uh, to detect cervical cancer or pre-cancer."

"Well, does the patient have a cervix?"

"No."

"Did she have a hysterectomy for cancer?"

"No."

"Then does she need a Pap?"

"No."

"You have answered your own question, grasshopper. Please call again."

"Wait, can I ask another question?"

"Why not?"

"Is it true that you don't need Paps after age 65?"

"That would be true. As long as the patient has had normal screening up to that point, she does not need Paps past that age."

"Wow, that's great, and this machine is great too, thanks."

"You're welcome, and thanks for using *First Call Interactive*."

Chapter 21

Receiving a Massage from a Man

I have not always been a fan of massage. It was not until I had been in practice for many years that I learned that one of life's greatest pleasures is massage. I had always thought about getting a massage when I was on vacation, but they were always more expensive at hotels and seemed self-indulgent. Also, do you need a massage while on vacation? You're already relaxed. You need a massage on a Wednesday afternoon when you are stressed out at work, checking on your 401k to see how soon you can retire. They should have massage therapists at work.

Actually, some progressive hospitals do provide massages at work. When I worked at a hospital in Fremont, California, they had one. Employers have found that a fifteen-minute massage for employees decreases stress and work-related accidents. The massage therapist at the Fremont hospital was a woman that was so strong I would hear cracking sounds and would ask her to ease up. I remember laying there prone on her massage table and wondering if I were to suffer a broken rib from the massage if it would be considered a work-related injury.

I thought I would try a massage school in my town called Triplet College. I didn't really need a professional massage—a trainee would be adequate, and I could save money. My wife can give an excellent massage and it is free. The only problem is that she loses interest after thirty seconds. As her interest in the massage wanes, her massage starts to slow down. I shout out, "More, more!" She speeds up for ten seconds and then says, "Done."

I called up Triplet College and asked, "Why are you called Triplet?" The receptionist responded, "Because we not only offer courses to become a certified massage therapist but also offer courses to become medical assistants and paralegals."

"Hmm," I jokingly replied, "Maybe you can teach me how to legally write off my massages for medical reasons." There was complete silence on the other end.

The receptionist then asked, "What kind of massage would you like?" I started to panic. I didn't want to sound like a novice. I said, "I would like a legitimate massage." I immediately regretted my answer. The receptionist replied that they only gave legitimate massages, and she suggested a Swedish massage. I quickly replied, "Yes, that's what I meant."

When I arrived, my massage therapist greeted me. He turned out to be a man! It had not occurred to me that I might have a male massage therapist. I don't mind having a male auto mechanic, but you feel more vulnerable when you are undressed. It turns out that most men and women prefer a female therapist, so if you don't give a preference, you are likely to receive a male therapist.

He said, "Hi, I'm Randy." I replied, "I'm sure you are." He asked me if there were any areas of my body I did not want to be massaged. All I could think of was, "My buttocks." He replied, "Alright, but massaging your 'glutes' is the best part of the massage." I thought, "Hmm," as my "glutes" tightened up.

During the massage, Randy's one-inch-long blond arm hair would brush up against my skin. That did not help me relax. He gave an excellent deep tissue massage, but I didn't feel comfortable getting a massage from a man. I have had many women tell me they feel the same way. Some women think a heterosexual male therapist may check out or judge their bodies, and a man worries that a homosexual male may be doing the same. Men are concerned that the male massage therapist may be gay. Women worry that he isn't.

My haircutter, Laura, told me that she once had a good-looking male massage therapist and felt she had to hold her abdomen in during the massage and then started to worry that the cellulite on her thighs was showing. She went on to say that this was not a problem with a female massage therapist, as most female therapists are heavier than she is.

Even though the massage is non-sexual, many men find a woman's touch to be more pleasant and relaxing. However, some men and women prefer a male therapist as they are stronger and give a better deep tissue massage.

I explained my preference for a female massage therapist to a friend of mine. She herself is a massage therapist. She said, "Do you know what your aversion to men touching you means?"

"No," I replied.

She continued, "It means that you are curious."

"Curious about what?"

"Curious about men."

"No, it doesn't!" I exclaimed.

"Well, aren't you just a little curious?"

I replied, "Well, maybe just a... No!"

Chapter 22

The French Laundry

The city of Fairfield, California, has grown significantly since 1982 when my family and I first moved here.

Like many towns in America, we have a big mall that has taken considerable business away from the downtown shopping area. The mall's name has since changed, but it was Westfield Shoppingtown Solano. Of course, nobody ever said, "Do you want to go to Westfield Shoppingtown Solano?" We just called it Solano Mall or the mall.

We have every chain of restaurants, as you can imagine, but we have very few excellent restaurants. Our local newspaper does a survey every year to inform us of the most popular businesses in town. Bryan-Braker has been the best funeral parlor for most years. Rockville Florist is often rated the best florist. Joe's Buffet has the best roast beef in town. Our Yellow Pages (if you can find a Yellow Pages) lists six McDonald's restaurants. One year the survey said the best place to have lunch was McDonald's. That statement sums up the restaurant situation in Fairfield.

We could use a few more ethnic restaurants in Fairfield. I wish we had more Korean, Vietnamese, Filipino, and Afghani restaurants.

We have three Denny's restaurants. Two of them are on the same block. When my nurse anesthetist friend John and I decide to go to breakfast at 6 am after a delivery, I always ask him if he wants to go to the one on Holiday Lane or the one on Holiday Lane. I have no idea why there are two Denny's on the same block.

When we want a perfect meal, we leave Fairfield and go to a little town in the Napa Valley called Yountville. It is a town of only several thousand people, but it has a half dozen of the best restaurants in California. My favorite restaurant is in what looks like a little house. It is called the French Laundry because the restaurant's stone building used to be a French steam laundry in the 1920s. I've eaten in several five-star restaurants, but none are better than this. We used to get the pharmaceutical salespeople to take us out for fine dining. The government has now put considerable restrictions on pharmaceutical dinners, so they don't take us to great restaurants anymore.

I recall one particular pharmaceutical company that took us to the French Laundry. We would tell the sales rep that we only used her brand of estrogen replacement pills — Premarin. Later, another company would take us to dinner, and we would tell them that we used their products exclusively. Meanwhile, we always wrote for generic drugs. The reps were on to us as they paid for data from the local pharmacies, but they played along. They were just happy that we did not kick them out when they entered our medical building, as many doctors do. They were pleased to have us as a captive audience. They believed that if they could tell us how superior their drugs were compared to their competitors, we would change our prescribing habits.

The dining experience at the French Laundry is nothing short of several hours of heavenly bliss. I have not been there in many years, so I don't know if they have changed their policy, but in the past, it took three months to get a reservation there for a Saturday night. I would call three months ahead, to the day. I had to call at 10 am. If I did not have a reservation by 10:20, I was not likely to get one.

If you are in a group, the food is brought out before it is prepared. The chef may bring out sea bass and tell you where it was caught. He may tell you everything about the sea bass except for the name of the fisherman who caught it. You will then learn how it will be prepared, and an appropriate wine will be suggested.

A dish called "Peas and Carrots" consists of a lobster pancake with pea shoot salad and ginger-carrot emulsion. I was a biology major, but I don't know what part of the pea the shoot is. Also, isn't an emulsion what you get when you mush things together? I guess ginger-carrot emulsion sounds better than ginger-carrot mush or ginger-carrot paste.

How would they describe mashed potatoes at the French Laundry? They might say: "An Irish-American classic made from a puree of the potato root."

How would they describe the salt that they grind onto the potato with a pepper mill? One could imagine them saying: "This Fleur de Sel Atlantic sea salt is harvested on a specific week in July when the perfect combination of humidity and sun form a bloom of white on the salt marshes of Brittany, France. We then allow the salt to crystallize slowly and unrefined in the wind, thus giving the salt a subtle hickory flavor. The flavor is bold but not pretentious. The same could not be said of our menu."

Another interesting dish is cleverly called Tongue in Cheek. It consists of braised beef cheeks and veal tongue with baby leaks and horseradish cream. I don't have the courage to try it, but one would have to assume that cheek meat is quite tender. Consider how soft your own cheeks are.

The courses keep coming at the French Laundry. The courses are small and dazzling, leaving you wanting more. Fortunately, the portions are small. How else would you be able to finish nine courses?

At the end of one of the courses, the waiter surprised us with a tiny ice cream cone filled with salmon tartar. It's much better than it sounds, but most remarkably, it was free!

The waiter described the butter that we were spreading on our bread. I think the story went something like this: "The butter comes from a woman who raises only three free-range cows in Orwell, Vermont that are massaged daily and given an organic diet. These cows make butter exclusively for the French Laundry. The salt that is added is imported and specially chosen for this butter. The butter is shipped overnight to the French Laundry.

I asked my wife what she thought of the butter. She said, "I can't believe it's not better." Those were my thoughts, exactly. It just tastes like butter. It tastes the same as the butter from a penned-up constipated cow that spends her day walking around in her own poop.

Not all my friends are as impressed as I am with the French Laundry. My friend Bob is a plastic surgeon. He says that eating there is a religious experience because when you get the bill, you say, "Jesus Christ!" Actually, the bill is not that outrageous, considering that this may be a once-in-a-lifetime experience. My son, however, pointed out that he could eat at Taco Bell for a year with what we paid for our dinner. Even though it is a bit pricey, you only go on special occasions, such as when someone else is paying.

My friend, Christian, is a frugal family doctor. He buys a whole chicken at the grocery store on Saturday and keeps eating it all week. By Friday, he has to eat the wings, and then he buys a new chicken. He says the portions at the French Laundry are too small considering the price. He calls it the French Cleaners.

Chapter 23

Touring Italy with Beatrice

Beatrice (pronounced Bee-ah-tree-che) is a rare jewel. She is a vibrant, short woman with a strong Italian accent. Beatrice was our tour guide for the eight days that we spent touring Italy. As our den mother, she told us when to wake up in the morning, which could be as early as 6:30 a.m. She told us about Italian customs so we wouldn't find ourselves in awkward situations. One such bit of advice was that we were to tip the attendant at public restrooms. That was to maintain the toilets in a state of cleanliness. Without this, the bathrooms would be like those at gas stations in the United States. The tips were often discretionary. It could be as little as thirty cents. My wife says that if you really have to go and don't have any change, they may let you go, anyway.

Some drives on the tour bus were rather long. Beatrice kept the ride enjoyable with amusing anecdotes. She also knew that we might like to take a nap in the comfortable air-conditioned motor coach, so she discreetly turned off her microphone and let us sleep after lunch. She gently woke us up if an interesting site came into view.

One day after lunch, we drove by what appeared to be a fourteenth-century castle. As people were napping, Beatrice did not comment. I was annoyed. We never see things similar to this in the U.S. Driving by without comment was like driving by the Loch Ness monster and saying nothing. Such wonders are commonplace in Europe.

Beatrice told us that women in Italy had gained more power in recent years. She worked full-time. "Women don't just stay home and have babies in Italy anymore," she said. "Women were given the vote in Italy in 1946. Unfortunately, aggressive women are being blamed for men becoming gay in Italy."

"Whoa, whoa, whoa," I said, "*Un momento per piacere*. It's going to take a lot more than a woman voting to turn me gay."

Beatrice agreed. She thought there had always been gay men in Italy, but only recently had so many felt comfortable coming out of the closet.

In front of the whole bus, she then asked me, "Matsumura, how do they treat women in Japan?" It immediately occurred to me that she thought that I was from Japan, and why not? I was the only Japanese on the bus, and I had a Nikon camera around my neck.

I replied in my best Italian accent, "Een my country… woman walk five feet behind man, but when I come to U.S., woman walk all over man." My fellow American travelers found this quite amusing, not because of my old joke, but because they all knew that I'm an American, and I don't know any more about Japan than they do.

As we drove back into Rome, Beatrice pointed out the prostitutes lining the main thoroughfare. I looked at my watch. It was only 4:40 in the afternoon. Beatrice explained that even though prostitution is illegal, the women of the night were trying to market themselves to the commuters on their way home. They wore high heels, low-cut blouses, very short miniskirts, and a lot of makeup. My children find museums to be very boring but this was not. Suddenly their noses were pressed against the windows, as was mine.

Beatrice then asked me, "Matsumura, what do they call prostitutes in Japan?" I had no idea, so I responded, "We call them *Signorinas de la notte*." Beatrice got a surprised look on her face and said, "That's what we call them here." I responded, "It's a universal profession."

As we were driving through beautiful Tuscany, Beatrice was reminded of a town she once tried to visit in Arizona with a similar name: Tucson.

She stopped at a gas station in Arizona to get directions but was told there was no such city named Tucson. She pronounced the "c" in Tucson just as one pronounces the "c" in Tuscany. She explained she was sure that she was in the correct state and pointed to Tucson on her map. The attendant laughed and explained that Tucson was pronounced with a silent "c."

Italians have watched many American movies, so while in Arizona, Beatrice rented a red convertible Mustang. What could be more American than that? While speeding outside Yuma, she was spotted by a patrolman who pulled up behind her with his lights flashing. Beatrice informed us that in Italy, the speed limit was more of a suggestion.

Beatrice ignored him, so he pulled up alongside her and signaled for her to pull over. She was the only car on the road, but she pointed to herself as if to say, "Who, me?"

She pulled over and spoke to him only in Italian even though she was fluent in English. He asked for her driver's license, so she pulled out her three full-page Italian driver's license. Frustrated, the patrolman showed Beatrice on the speedometer the maximum allowable speed. She gave a nod of understanding. He let her go without giving her a ticket.

Chapter 24

Wall $treet Week

If you are younger than age fifty, you may not remember a show on public television that was mostly about the stock market. It was called *Wall Street Week* with Louis Rukeyser. It aired every Friday night for thirty-two years. It was the most popular financial show of its time, by far.

My children would hear the familiar intro music come on at the beginning of the show and call me to watch.

Lou's program started way before one could turn to the internet or CNBC for up-to-the-minute financial information. When it came to credibility, he was the Walter Cronkite of financial news. We viewers were saddened when Lou passed away from cancer. Michael Holland, a frequent guest on the show, said that no one could replace him. An attempt was made to replace Lou, but the ratings collapsed, and the show was canceled. Although I miss the end of the week wrap-up of the market, I'm glad the show was canceled, as it would not have been the same without Lou.

Holland also said, "He brought financial journalism to a new level with his trademarks of honesty, humor, and fairness. He always looked at both sides of the issue. His only bias was toward optimism."

I liked to call him Uncle Lou. I'm not sure how good an investment guru he was. He seemed to be perpetually bullish on the market, but then so are most successful investment celebrities. Uncle Lou enjoyed a good market, but one got the feeling that he enjoyed a good pun even more.

He once answered a letter on the air about investing in a hairpiece producer. He smiled as he said, "If your money seems to be hair today and gone tomorrow, we'll try to make it grow back by giving you the bald facts on how to get your investments toupee."

My wife, who is not interested in Wall Street, would watch him just to observe his dry humor and to see him wink. I think part of his longevity on television can be attributed to him not taking himself too seriously.

I remember watching Lou's show on October 16, 1987. His first guest that night was the late Martin Zweig, whose self-effacing manner made him most likable. Zweig said in that interview, "I've been really, in my own mind, looking for a crash, but I didn't want to talk about it publicly because it's like shouting 'fire' in a crowded theater and there are other ways to play it."

The following Monday, October 19, 1987, became known as Black Monday. The market dropped 22% in a single day. That was the largest single-day drop ever, even lower than any day in 1929. It was the most prescient call I had ever witnessed. Marty, as Lou called him, said not to panic, as the pain would only last a few months. Sure enough, by the end of the year, the market had recovered.

Uncle Lou continued to work into his seventies. Could it be that he forgot to plan for retirement, so he had to keep working? Obviously, he just loved his work.

Off and on, I would subscribe to his newsletter. Several times a year, I would make a purchase of a stock based on his recommendation. Of those purchases, I don't recall ever losing money on a trade. On the other hand, it was difficult to lose money in the great bull market that ended in the tech bubble that burst in 2000. Despite the good recommendations, I would often let my newsletter subscription run out.

Uncle Lou didn't like to lose a subscriber. He would send me complimentary copies of the newsletter, hoping to get me back. He pleaded with me, telling me how I was one of his original charter subscribers. Now that Uncle Lou was wealthy, he had not forgotten his friends who had supported him when he was a mere millionaire.

He kept sending me letters, discounting the annual price of the newsletter. Apparently, this special offer was only for me because the renewal form was not transferable. Did Uncle Lou really think I was going to fall for such sappy marketing? If Uncle Lou is in heaven reading this, his answer would be, "You betcha," as he gives his trademark wink.

Chapter 25

Thai Food

I have an obstetrical colleague named Julie. Julie is Chinese. She and I have found that when we are very busy in the labor and delivery suite, that is a good time to order Thai food, as no one has time to go down to the cafeteria. An even better time to order Thai food is when we are not busy.

Our routine goes like this. Someone suggests that we get Thai food. The nurses and doctors all choose one dish, and then we eat family style. I like the Pad Thai noodles. Julie usually orders Tom Kha soup. The waiter who takes the order always asks, "How hot you want?" We always ask for the food to be extra hot (spicy hot, not temperature hot), but it usually doesn't come back hot enough for Julie. Now we have Julie order because we find that when she orders, with her Chinese accent, the food comes back much hotter.

One day one of the OB nurses told Julie that she wanted to order the soup of the day, which she said was Cream of Sum Yung Gai. This, of course, is a joke. Although Julie has a fairly good command of the English language, she does not understand the subtlety of some jokes.

Julie called in the order by phone. Soon she called out to the nurse, "They don't have soup of today, and they don't have Cream of Sum Yung Gai." A patient who was registering near the phone smiled.

Julie and I like Tom Kha soup. It comes with chicken, mushrooms, and lemongrass in a coconut milk broth. It is so good it should be called Tom Yum soup. There actually is a Thai soup with that name.

We have to order more than one order of soup because people like it at varying degrees of spiciness. Julie orders it extra hot because she likes it that way. I drink her extra hot soup so I can look like a man in front of all the nurses. This doesn't work out so well because I end up wiping away my tears for most of the meal. It burns, but it burns in a good way. You really know you are alive when you drink this soup. I could not track the exact path of my esophagus in my chest until I tried Julie's soup. I've wondered if you couldn't make a similar soup by combining one part of chicken broth with one part of Tabasco. Sometimes we call it "burn you twice soup."

Julie always says the same thing when she drinks her soup, "This soup isn't hot enough. I've had hotter than this. Why didn't they make it hotter?" She says this as she wipes the perspiration from her brow.

A few of the nurses are from the Midwest and find Thai food to be too exotic for their liking, but they don't want to feel left out. One such nurse is Lee. If Lee eats anything spicier than ketchup, she says, "Ooh, ooh," as she fans her open mouth with her open hand. For Lee, we order a special dish on the menu. It is called Citrus

Chicken. It is basically just Kentucky Fried Chicken that comes with a sauce, but we let her think she is eating something exotic. For her, we affectionately call it: "White Girl Chicken."

Chapter 26

Procardia XL

I was driving home from the office when I received a call from the pharmacist at Raley's— a grocery store that also has a pharmacy. This was back in the day before we prescribed medications electronically on the computer. The pharmacist told me that he had an irate patient in front of him who was trying to fill one of my prescriptions.

It just so happened that I was driving home, and I was about to pass this Raley's so I told the pharmacist to tell the patient to wait for five minutes and I would straighten everything out.

The patient was surprised to see me walk into the pharmacy a few minutes later. She told me she had been given a piece of paper at her last office visit that had said Sutter Health strived to exceed her expectations, but she didn't think it was actually true.

I smiled and told her, "We are Sutter, and this is how we roll."

She smiled and said, "That would make a good slogan. What is your current Sutter slogan?

I replied, "I'm not sure. I think it's something like: *Sutter Health, we're not so bad.* No, actually it is *Sutter*

Health, With You for Life." "You mean like herpes?" she joked.

I had written a refill prescription for this patient, Ms. Grover. I normally would prescribe a generic drug, but this particular drug had not yet become available generically. The name of the drug was Procardia XL. The patient tried to fill the prescription, but the pharmacist had refused.

I asked the pharmacist, "What's the problem?"

He explained, "The patient's insurance doesn't cover that drug." "Well," I replied, "does her insurance cover Adalat CC?"

"Yes, it does," said the pharmacist.

"Well, then why didn't you just substitute the Adalat CC 60 mg for the Procardia XL 60 mg?" I asked with some aggravation.

He came back with, "Well, we can't do that without a new written or verbal prescription from you."

"Why not?" I asked. "The generic name for both of them is nifedipine. They are both extended-release forms and are dosed once a day. They are both the same drug, aren't they?

The pharmacist replied, "Well…I can't say that."

"Why can't you say that?"

"Because I'm not allowed to say that the same drug made by two different companies under two proprietary names are exactly the same."

"Really, even though the generic name is the same and the milligram strength is the same and they are both taken once a day?"

"Exactly."

"On the other hand, if this was available as a generic drug, you could fill either brand name with a generic made by any number of different companies, right?"

"Right."

I went on, "You could fill it even though the generic may not have the exact same potency strength milligram for milligram, right?"

"Well, I can't say that," replied the pharmacist.

"Never mind," said I. "We won't go there. I guess there could be subtle differences in the long-acting part of the drug. Would you please substitute the Procardia XL with Adalat CC?"

"Sure, no problem, Dr. Matsumura."

The patient, at this point, looked very pleased. "Well, Dr. Matsumura," she says, "I appreciate you coming over here personally to straighten this out."

I laughed and said, "You know what we say, *'Sutter Health, With You for Life, as long as you don't lose your insurance.'*"

Chapter 27

A Frugal Flyer Tries Business Class

Around the time I was completing my residency training in Los Angeles, I came across a travel agent in my local mall. Yes, it used to be commonplace to see travel agents in malls. It is difficult to imagine now, but prior to the internet, one would go to a brick-and-mortar store to book tours and airline tickets. At the travel agent's store, I obtained a brochure from Eastern Airlines offering a twenty-one-day unlimited mileage fare that allowed one to fly anywhere they flew for $320. Kathy and I did not have that kind of cash, but we did have a credit card. I think I earned about $36,000 per year, which was adequate to live on in those days. I dreamed of seeing historic Boston, the pyramids of Yucatan, Mexico, and island hopping in the Caribbean. I remember how excited I was when I showed Kathy the brochure. Kathy said she could not think of any reason not to buy the pass.

We had so little money in those days. In Ocho Rios, Jamaica, we went to the market where the locals shopped. We bought cheese and bread—which we then ate in our hotel room–but we felt we were living the good life. We were jetsetters. With every meal, Eastern Airlines gave us a small bottle of wine. We didn't drink, so we would stash the bottles in our carry-on luggage. We would later give the wine to friends.

Through the years, I would on occasion see other airlines offer unlimited international flight passes for a fixed price. In my career, I never had the luxury of time to be able to take advantage of those deals. I did read about a man who did. He was enjoying his trip around the world, stopping at all the destinations on his bucket list. But one night he woke up on a plane in a momentary panic. He sat up in his seat and couldn't remember which city he had just left or where he was going.

In those days, we would fly in the economy section, and we were grateful to be there. We assumed the first-class section was for people traveling on business with a corporate expense account.

Flash forward forty years. Having a successful practice, I had considerably more disposable income than I did as a resident. I had completed a wonderful, escorted tour of Croatia and was finishing my vacation with a side trip to Germany. I was taking a three-hour Third Reich walking tour in Munich when a text message came over my phone from Lufthansa Airlines. I was being offered an upgrade from economy to business class for my trip home for an extra $1,200. I don't like to waste money, so I thought about it long and hard. I even went through the exercise of figuring out it would cost me about $100 extra per hour to upgrade. I proposed the following to myself: Would I be willing to sit in an uncomfortable seat for twelve hours if paid $100 per hour to do so? If I would, then I should decline the upgrade.

I probably would be willing to sit in that uncomfortable seat for that price. When I was younger, I would take an OB/GYN call for $100 per hour. But then I remembered that I am a lung cancer survivor (more on that later), and I may not live long enough to spend all of my retirement nest egg, so I may as well buy the upgrade. I knew I was rationalizing to get a good seat. The longer I thought about those cramped economy seats, the more I leaned toward the promotion. I quickly responded yes on my smartphone before I had time to change my mind. Up to that point, I had not been looking forward to flying home. For me, the only unpleasant part of an overseas vacation is flying to the destination and back.

I recalled flying in business class once before. I was checking in with the airlines on my computer the night before a trip to Hawaii. The airlines offered me an upgrade to premium economy where my family of four would all have extra legroom if I just paid $50 more per person. I upgraded all of our seats. When we arrived at the check-in counter the next day, the lady told us that the plane we would be departing on did not have premium economy seats, and our previous seats, which had all been together, had now been given to other passengers so we would all have to sit separately. The airline employee looked at my wife and could see that her face was turning red with anger. The employee knew the next words out of my wife's mouth were not going to be pleasant, so the employee solved the problem without even discussing it with us. She said, "Wow, look at this. You have all just received free upgrades to business class. Three of you will be sitting next to each other in the back row of the business class section and you, Mr. Matsumura, will be sitting by yourself near the front."

Halfway across the Pacific Ocean, my wife came up to use the restroom near where I was sitting. I asked her why she didn't just use the restrooms in the economy section, which were just one row behind her. She said, "You don't expect me to share the restroom with those in the cheap seats do you?" We both laughed.

I arrived at Frankfurt Airport two hours early for my trip home to San Francisco. The line for the checking-in of economy passengers was about eighty people long. The line for business and first-class passengers was empty, yet there was a female attendant there to guide me down the path of privilege.

I thought the whole walk of pride thing was interesting, so I took a picture of the contrasting lines to show my wife later. Suddenly, out of nowhere, an employee of the airport came out and told me in a German accent, "Picture-taking is not allowed in the check-in area!" Since I am of Asian descent, I smiled, pretended I did not speak English, and said, "Gomen'nasai," which I think means sorry in Japanese. I bowed slightly. She gave me a weak smile and walked away. I thought, inappropriately, she is probably the descendant of a Gestapo agent.

I made my way to the executive lounge, where I found a lady there at the entrance who keeps out the riffraff. That would normally be me.

My first stop would be the dining section. Although I had a full buffet breakfast in my hotel just two hours earlier, I decided to have some eggs and potatoes since it was "free." I noticed that they had every imaginable bottle of alcohol in their well-stocked bar. There was even beer on tap.

I saw a man drinking hard liquor at 10:00 am. I thought, "Well, it must be 5 pm somewhere—probably where he just flew in from."

This stylish man was wearing a tan scarf around his neck and appeared to be carrying a matching purse. He looked up and saw me staring at him just as I was stuffing a complimentary bottle of juice into my carry-on bag. Since he saw me, I smiled and winked at him. He smiled and winked back.

"Oh my God," I said to myself. "What have I just done? I hope he doesn't think I'm attracted to him." I quickly got up and left the dining section of the lounge and moved to an overstuffed chair.

From there, I could see a wall of complimentary newspapers available, but few were in English. One was called *Die Welt*. I took a *New York Times*. I would have preferred the easier-to-read and superficial *USA Today*, but they didn't have any.

I noticed that they had showers available. Near the shower area was a woman who appeared to have a full-time job cleaning the restrooms.

The cleaning lady seats you. Well, she doesn't seat you, but she directs you to a cleaned restroom. It is not just a stall, but a small room with four walls that go all the way from the floor to the ceiling for your hygienic privacy. I usually dread public restrooms because they are often dirty and not very private. I thought, "This is the life. If I am ever homeless, this is where I would like to stay, although gaining access to this lounge may be problematic."

Earlier, when I was looking for this executive lounge, I was in a different part of the airport and had tried to gain entrance to the Lufthansa first-class lounge. I was told that in Frankfurt, the business class lounge is separate from the first-class lounge. I needed to find the business-class lounge and was given directions. That got me thinking, "What could they possibly have in the first-class lounge that is not in the business-class lounge?" The first thing that came to mind was that they had an attendant in the restroom who gives men that final shake when they are done urinating. Actually, now I have to give my penis a shake, another shake, and then two dabs with a tissue. I wish that I could wring it out like a sponge. This dribbling problem has been happening to me since I turned sixty—very annoying. I wonder if I could solve the problem with a clothespin.

I thought, maybe the first-class lounge has eggs that can be custom ordered. "I would like my eggs over-easy, Fritz."

First-class can be twice as expensive as business class. Some airlines are getting rid of first-class because the cost is so prohibitive that few can afford it. Reportedly Singapore Airlines offers Dom Perignon with caviar, and that is before takeoff.

The Lufthansa first-class lounge in Frankfurt may be quite far from your departing gate. If that is the case, I am told, they will drive you to your plane in a Porsche or Mercedes.

Can first-class ever be "over the top?" Consider Etihad Airways. They offer a three-room suite with a permanent double bed in the bedroom, a living room, and a private bathroom with a shower. You have access to an onboard chef, and there is a nanny to help take care of your children. When I checked the price, a ticket from New York to Abu Dhabi was $32,000.

Before paying for an upgraded seat, one may want to go online and see what one is paying for. Domestic United States business class seats are only a bit nicer than flying coach, also known as economy class. The same airline can have different levels of business class, even on the same model jetliner.

Finally, I boarded the plane. Business class is in the front of the aircraft, and we were allowed to board early. That forced all the other passengers to have to do their walk of shame past us as they shuffled to the back of the plane to their cramped lower-class seats. As they passed, they saw us drinking champagne out of crystal glasses. They probably wondered what we were celebrating. We were celebrating the fact that we didn't have to sit in coach.

The plane took off. That is the point where I usually fall asleep. I believe I fall asleep at that point because on taxiing out to the runway, the plane's fumes enter the cabin and drug the passengers. Then, on takeoff, the seats are reclined due to the angle of the ascent.

This time, I decided to force myself to stay awake as I didn't want to miss any of the business-class amenities. Sure enough, once we leveled off, they started to serve us lunch. I was now eating my third meal in six hours.

I later learned that you could eat your meals at your convenience and not at designated times.

The flight attendants bring your food on trays that they carry to your seat just as you would be served in a restaurant. That may seem like a little thing, but by not using that large pushcart, the aisle is not blocked, so there is always access to the restroom.

After lunch, I decided to recline my seat, which could go all the way flat if I so desired. I decided to recline a bit and watch a movie. I caught the flight attendant's attention and complained to her that the touch screen was too far away for me to reach. A smile came across her face as she handed me my remote control.

Like many Americans, I am concerned about income inequality in our country. The rich are very rich, and the middle class can't seem to get ahead. This can lead to social unrest. When the economic concerns of the people are ignored, populist movements can take root. Hitler came to power when he gave the German people hope from the economic despair they faced after World War I.

If the revolution ever comes, I picture it starting in the economy section of a plane as they overthrow the aristocracy sitting in business class.

I can picture a young militant Bernie Sanders' supporter (such as my daughter) waking up on a long flight. She is cranky and sticky after having a fitful sleep sitting upright for the last ten hours. She tries to reach for her magazine, but she can't reach it. It is stowed behind the seat in front of her, but that seat is in her face.

She now peers through the sheer curtain that separates business class from economy and sees that we are receiving hot washcloths. Next, she sees us eating coconut and fresh mango oatmeal with chia seeds on china with real silverware.

When she sees me wiping my mouth with a white cloth napkin, she decides she can't take it anymore. She incites her fellow passengers to storm our section of the plane. Our flight attendants set up a barricade of extra thick blankets and empty wine bottles. I ask my flight attendant what all the commotion is about. She informs me that the peasants in the economy section have no bread. I tell her, "Let them eat peanuts."

Usually, I am very parsimonious, which in my case is a euphemism for just being cheap. I was raised in a poor family and can't seem to get that out of my system. Even though I am a physician, I buy all of my cars for half price by buying them used. I wanted to replace my twenty-year-old, light, waterproof, Faconnable jacket but found that a new one would cost me $500. I found a used one on the internet for $25. (I told my friend, Dr. Katz, about this Faconnable deal. He asked if there were any more Faconnable jackets available for $25. I told him no and now he says he hates me.) At one time, I tried cutting my own hair to save money. I had to give that up when someone asked me if I cut my own hair.

When I was young, I would notice people were traveling business class, but it never occurred to me to upgrade as the price of an upgrade could pay for a whole new vacation. Back then it was exciting enough to be going overseas.

I have never received such attentive and deferential service as when flying business class. I was made to feel as though I was king for a day. I would swear that the 11.5-hour trip only took 6 hours.

I know I have waxed on about the benefits of traveling business class, but it isn't really about how great business class is. It is about how terrible the alternative is — sitting in the economy section. It seems to me that those seats have been getting smaller through the years, which makes no sense, as we are getting larger. If the person in front of you reclines, you will have no legroom. I am relatively short. How do tall people fit in those seats? Basically, in the economy section, you are cattle.

If you fly economy, your trip becomes about the destination and not the journey. If you fly business class, you can savor the journey.

I know that I will continue to be frugal with all my other purchases, but if I am going to travel overseas, I no longer consider business class a luxury. It is a necessity. At my age, if I can't afford to go business class, I'll just have to keep saving my money or not go at all.

Chapter 28

Weed Whacker

We bought a house on five acres of land when I was twenty-nine years old. I thought it would be great to have a large estate so that we could keep up with the Joneses. Who are the Joneses? They are an imaginary professional couple that lives on a large estate in our neighborhood. The wife drives a Range Rover, and her husband drives an all-electric Porsche. The wife is the CFO of a Napa winery and her husband is a financial advisor. They both went to Yale and somehow manage to work that into every conversation. They never actually mention Yale. They say, "Back in New Haven we used to…." Unfortunately, the Joneses met their demise when their cigarette boat was hit by a rogue wave.

I too wanted to someday live the country club lifestyle. When we first moved into our home, I drove a 1971 Plymouth Duster, but hoped to trade it in as we became more upwardly mobile. Our winding driveway was very long. We had a great view of the San Francisco East Bay Area. I jokingly called our home Rancho Matsumura.

I did not realize how much work it would be to maintain a large property even though most of our land was undeveloped chaparral. The two acres of land in front of our house had weeds that would dry out and become a fire hazard.

Each year, for the last thirty years, I would decide to cut down the weeds myself when the rains stopped in late spring. It gave me a feeling of accomplishment to do some manual labor. People would ask me if I had a gardener. I would say, "Yes, I have a Japanese gardener — me."

Some of the star thistle weeds have stems (or should I say trunks) that are one inch thick. I would cut right through them with a thick nylon cord attached to a gasoline-powered weed whacker. You have to get these weeds while they are still green. If you wait until they are brown and dry, they don't cut away as easily. It takes a full-time worker about five days to cut down all the weeds.

After a long day of weed cutting (about two hours), I looked like an actor from the *Texas Chain Saw Massacre* movie. The difference was that I had green plant "blood" all over my face and glasses.

I would struggle back up the hill to the house, dragging the weed whacker behind me. I explained to my wife that the novelty of weed-whacking had worn off and we would have to hire someone to cut the rest of the weeds. She reassured me that she had already hired someone.

We would then both go outside to look down the hill to assess how much of the weeds I had cut down. At first, we couldn't find where I had been working. The weeds couldn't possibly have grown back that fast. Then my wife would spot the area. She would say, "There it is. It looks like you cut the postage stamp out of a large letter."

"Yes," I would beam, "I did that myself."

Fortunately, there are quite a few migrant workers in our area that work in the local fruit orchards and wineries. These workers would often come to our house and ask if they could cut down the weeds. They would start approaching us in the early spring, but the weeds were still growing at that time, so my wife turned them away. I taught my wife to tell them, "*Regresa el uno de Mayo*," which means, "Return the first of May."

My wife had trouble telling these workers apart. She thought it was just one worker who kept calling on her for work every few weeks and she kept telling him to return on May 1. On May 1, we had a small army reporting for duty.

We noticed that these day laborers were getting more sophisticated. It used to be that we would hire a worker and he would arrive by bicycle. Our last worker had a van, a smartphone, and business cards. He is a Mexican who subcontracted other Mexicans to work for him.

Weed whackers (the machines) are very temperamental and break down frequently if you have a jungle to cut down. One day the migrant worker, Alex, brought back the weed whacker to my wife to report that it was not working properly. He wanted to tell her that the machine needed repair, but he only spoke a little English. He said, "Lady, your machine…your machine is f**ked up." My wife wanted to start laughing but did not want Alex to think she was laughing at him, so she kept a straight face. She thinks she can speak Spanish by simply adding an "o" to English words. She said to Alex, "No problemo, mi esposo will fixo."

After forty years in that home, Kathy and I were aging, so we decided to downsize and move to a smaller house in town. We wanted a house that was much more manageable. We now live in a normal-sized suburban home. We no longer have to deal with the acres of weeds that have become a significant fire hazard in Northern California.

We no longer have rattlesnakes terrorizing us with their rattling sounds outside our bedroom window as we are trying to go to sleep. We no longer have deer destroying our garden. We used to have a well for our water supply, but the water was so full of iron we had to drink bottled water. We had no cable television. In our new home, we have fast internet and hundreds of TV programs, as well as movies we can stream.

Who knew the middle class had it so good? We should never have tried to keep up with the Joneses. Every day we remark on how great it is to live in our normal home.

Chapter 29

Premarin

What's in a word? I have to admit that I had prescribed Premarin for many years before realizing that PREMARIN was derived from the words: PREgnant MARes urINe. That's right, pregnant mare's urine—not that there's anything wrong with that.

Let me back up a moment. Premarin is the brand name of a hormone that many women use for estrogen replacement. Some women take estrogen to get rid of hot flashes when they go through menopause. Other women take it if, for some reason, they had their ovaries removed at a young age. These women usually want to replace the estrogen that their ovaries would have been making.

If you had been on estrogen replacement therapy before the year 2000, you were most likely taking Premarin or one of its related products such as Prempro.

There are quite a few brands of estrogen on the market. None of the others are made from horse urine. Some of the other brands are synthesized from yams and other plant sources. You can't, however, just eat yams and get the benefits of taking estrogen.

One might ask why patients would take something from horses' urine when there are plant-derived alternatives. Well, for one thing, Premarin has held most of the "shelf space" for the last forty years. If you go to the store to buy soup, you usually will find an abundance of the Campbell's brand. In the days when cameras used film, you could always find the Kodak brand. That doesn't necessarily mean those are the best brands, but they are the standards.

I had a patient who found out her Premarin was from horse urine and asked if I would switch her to something more "natural." I told her that horse's urine was very natural. She told me that it really didn't bother her knowing it was from horses, but she had read that the horses were confined to small stalls instead of running free, which bothered her.

Premarin had for many years been in the top five of the most prescribed medications in the U.S. It has become less popular as hormone replacement in light of concerns regarding its side effects.

After so many decades of being on the market, one has to wonder why someone has not come out with a generic substitute. After all, if you are prescribed Vicodin, Keflex, or Prozac, you will most likely get a generic substitute and not the brand name. Your prescription for a generic drug could cost less than $5.

As I understand it, the reason there is no substitute for Premarin is that for many years, no one knew exactly what was in Premarin. The estrogens in Premarin are called equine or horse estrogens. Now we know almost all the components of Premarin, but we still aren't sure what all the components do. You can't really call some of the minor chemicals in Premarin contaminants because, for all we know, these chemicals may enhance the medication's effects. Some doctors believe that Premarin is a better estrogen than the other synthesized estrogens.

The equine estrogens apparently work well for horses. They don't complain of hot flashes.

Chapter 30

Surrogate Mothers

I have had several infertile women seek out a surrogate mother to have their baby for them. Usually, the negotiating has been professionally done with lawyers involved. My first job is to sort out who the biological mother and biological father are.

Sometimes the surrogate mother is using her own eggs. When possible, the surrogate may be impregnated with the mother's fertilized egg who will be adopting the baby. In this case, the surrogate is acting as an incubator. She has no genetic connection to the baby. It can get confusing. I don't even want to think about the insurance implications.

Once I had sisters as patients. I walked into the exam room and was greeted by two women. One sister, Sydney, was going to have a baby for her infertile sister. I immediately made up a mnemonic to help me remember who was going to be delivering the kid. The mnemonic was, "Syd is the genetic mother of the kid."

Cheryl's ovaries had stopped working prematurely. Syd had been inseminated with the sperm of Cheryl's husband, Bill. Syd was the genetic mother, as Cheryl was not able to be an egg donor.

I examined Syd in the exam room. We listened to the baby's reassuring heartbeat. I asked Syd to get dressed and then asked the two sisters to meet with me in my office.

"Wow," I thought as I walked back to my office. Although I had not yet met Bill, I wondered how he felt about having a child with Syd. How would Syd feel someday when she came to visit? She would be seeing her own child living with relatives. How would Cheryl feel as the "mother?" She was the only player in this process that wasn't a first-degree relative of her child. She was actually the aunt of the child. What if Syd came over to visit and was giving advice on how to raise the child? Cheryl might say, "You have no right to come over here and tell me how to raise my child just because you are her actual mother."

Soon, Cheryl and Syd entered my office and sat down. I looked at Cheryl and asked if she could feel the baby move yet. She gave me a puzzled look and then replied, "Well…yes." I immediately realized my mistake. Now that they were both wearing clothes and in a different room, I had gotten the two of them mixed up. Fortunately, they forgave me. Moving on quickly, I asked my next question. Did they have attorneys and psychological counselors involved? They assured me that they did.

Surrogacy situations can be quite varied. I am aware of one case where a woman became a surrogate to carry her grandchild because her daughter had had a hysterectomy. I am never judgmental. These situations are never a patient's first choice.

As previously mentioned, surrogate adoptions are done professionally, or so I thought. Jennifer was a twenty-two-year-old Caucasian woman and had already had three healthy children from her previous boyfriend. She felt she was blessed with fertility and wanted to share her good fortune with an infertile couple. Jennifer knew an infertile married couple. The infertile woman was Caucasian, and her husband was Asian. Jennifer had decided to be a surrogate for the infertile couple and saw me for the first time while she was in labor. She had decided not to seek prenatal care, as her previous pregnancies had been uncomplicated (definitely not recommended).

I was nervous about this case as Jennifer was on welfare and had not sought out prenatal, legal, or psychological counseling. No legal documents had yet been drawn up.

I asked Jennifer how she had become pregnant, and she replied, "With a turkey baster."

Alright, so I could see that she had become pregnant at home with artificial insemination. As I left the labor room to write out my history, my head was swimming with the implications of what I had just heard.

I re-told the story to the labor nurse that would be caring for this patient. I told the nurse I was concerned that this baby was going to come out half black and half white, but the adopting parents were expecting a baby that was half white and half Asian. You see, the surrogate's boyfriend was black, and I was concerned that she and her boyfriend might have had sex near the time of the insemination, and then who knows what would be the outcome?

The young nurse was shocked when I told her about the turkey baster. Many years ago, turkey basters were commonly used by potential parents at home, but artificial insemination is now almost always done in the doctor's office. I told the nurse that turkey basters should come with the following instructions:

For artificial insemination: 1. Obtain consultation from an OB/GYN physician or, at the very least, carefully follow the instructions and understand how an ovulation kit works. 2. Obtain fresh semen specimen in a clean cup. 3. Carefully draw up semen and deposit it high in the vagina at the time of ovulation. 4. Wash the baster thoroughly before placing back in the drawer.

Anyway, two hours later, the baby was delivered, and it looked like an Anglo-Asian baby. After the delivery, I went back to the nurse's station to do my paperwork. The nurses were anxious to learn of my findings. "It's an Anglo-Asian baby," I said.

One of the nurses asked, "How could you tell it was an Asian baby as opposed to a black baby? Did he have a small penis?" I was totally shocked by that question. My jaw dropped. I looked up and immediately realized that the nurses had set me up for this joke. They were laughing hysterically. I told them I was going to have to turn them all in for sexual harass…. I was laughing too hard to finish my sentence.

Chapter 31

Wrong Site Surgery

The following case occurred in 1995 to Willie King, a 52-year-old father of three. Mr. King had insulin-dependent diabetes that had become quite progressive. His peripheral disease was such that he had decreased blood circulating in his lower legs and decreased feeling. It is easy for people with diabetes this advanced to cut their foot and yet not feel it. The cut can then get infected, but the body has decreased ability to fight off the infection. This can lead to gangrene and ultimately amputation.

That was the situation here. The right foot and right lower leg were going to have to be amputated. Mr. King was admitted to a hospital in Tampa, Florida.

Unfortunately for Mr. King, the operating room computer printout mistakenly noted that he was to have a left-sided amputation. All hospitals ask the patient before surgery on which side they are going to be operated on. This was done by a nurse, and Mr. King correctly stated that it was the right lower leg. He jokingly added, "You know which one it is, don't you? I don't want to wake up and find the wrong one gone!" He was reassured.

In those days, in all surgical suite hallways, there was a large whiteboard announcing which patient would be in each room and what procedure was to be performed. Of course, this information was taken from the printed surgery schedule. The error was then transferred to the board. Surgeons would always look at this board before entering the operating room.

The surgeon must have glanced at the board, and soon the amputation was underway. During the case, a nurse reviewed the chart and noted that it was the right leg that was supposed to be operated on. She was crying as she told the surgeon, but it was too late. The surgeon saw Mr. King after the operation. He told King that he had removed his left leg. King said, "I thought we were going to do the right." The surgeon replied, "That's right, but we removed the left."

The right leg still needed amputation, so that surgery would have to be done. King had his right leg amputated at a different hospital.

The surgeon later tried to defend himself by saying that the left leg also had significant peripheral vascular disease and would eventually have needed amputation, anyway. The left leg did have significant disease, but it was still an egregious mistake. The *Wall Street Journal* reported the story under the title: "A Story That Doesn't Have a Leg to Stand On."

Many sympathetic colleagues came to the operating surgeon's defense. They said they would have likely made the same mistake given the same circumstances.

Two years later, Mr. King's surgeon would get into trouble again. While still on probation for his error in

Mr. King's case, he properly placed a catheter in a chest vein of a patient, but he placed it in the wrong patient.

The surgeon entered the correct room but then performed the surgery on the patient's roommate. The surgeon tried to blame the nurse who led him to the wrong patient and prepared the wrong patient for the procedure. It is prevalent to rely on the nurses for patient identification, but the surgeon is still ultimately responsible for checking the patient's nametag before starting the procedure. The surgeon was reprimanded with the following statement: "You can delegate, but you cannot delegate responsibility." The surgeon was placed on probation for another two years.

In 1996, at the same hospital where Mr. King had his surgery, a forty-two-year-old patient would have a healthy disk in his neck removed instead of his herniated disk. This later resulted in a lawsuit against the surgeon.

In one survey, twenty percent of a group of surgeons admitted that they had at least once operated on the wrong site.

Some surgeons used a felt-tip marker to place an "X" to mark the spot where the surgery would take place to avoid such errors. Unfortunately, sometimes the operating room tech would misinterpret this "X" to mean don't operate here. The tech might then ignore that side and prepare the other side for surgery by shaving and cleaning the "wrong" site.

Long ago, I decided I would put my initials on the surgical site. Currently, in all U.S. hospitals, there is a "time out" taken just before the beginning of the case to confirm that the surgeon is operating on the correct site and doing the correct procedure on the correct patient.

I once had to take a patient to surgery because she had an abscess (pus pocket) on the right side of her vulva, which was the size of a grapefruit. We took our time out, and the nurse asked me which side I would operate on. I told her it was the right side. It would have been impossible to operate on the left side, as the right side totally blocked access to the left, but it was still an essential exercise to go through.

Chapter 32

Reading Glasses

Something happened to me when I was in my forties — my vision got worse. I asked my cousin Wayne, who is an optometrist, what happened. He said, "You got old." I wasn't ready to admit I needed reading glasses. To read the newspaper, I would have to look over my glasses and bring the page to within four inches of my nose. One day I was doing an episiotomy repair while looking over my glasses. One of the nurses walked in and later remarked that I was so close to the episiotomy site that she thought I was kissing it. I told her that would be highly unlikely, considering all the blood and stool down there after a delivery.

It was very depressing. I had always thought you had to be seventy years old before you started buying *Reader's Digest* with the large print.

While at the pharmacy one day, I noticed some reading lenses that I could clip onto my glasses that only cost $10. Suddenly I could see many things that I had never noticed before, such as how much gray hair my wife had. For the first time, I also noticed I was growing a small forest of hair near my ear canals.

The problem with my clip-on lenses was that they made me look like I had a part in the movie *Revenge of the Nerds*. I was literally wearing glasses over my glasses. My kids started making fun of me and called me "six eyes." I soon got even with them — I started wearing them when I greeted their friends at the door.

My cousin Wayne said he could fix me up and have lenses placed in the bottom part of my regular glasses. They would be bifocals, but the line wouldn't show. I couldn't wait to get my new glasses. Finally, the anticipated day came, and I drove to his office to pick them up. I put them on and immediately looked for something to read. I found his bill and almost fell over. I exclaimed, "I only paid $500 for my first used car. It was a '71 Buick Electra that had factory air, electric windows, AM radio and could sleep four comfortably in the trunk." Wayne responded, "Well, you wanted transitional lenses so they could turn into sunglasses when you went outdoors. You wanted anti-scratch and anti-glare coatings. You wanted high-density lenses so you wouldn't look like you were wearing lenses as thick as Coke bottles. You wanted designer frames, and of course, you now have special progressive reading lenses in addition to your regular refracting lenses. And, I almost forgot, it comes with this free genuine faux-leather case."

Life is good now that I have my new glasses. The only complaint I have is that I can no longer lean back into the headrest when I drive my car. If I do, everything becomes a blur except for the bugs on the windshield, which come into perfect focus. I can now tell if a fly on the windshield is circumcised.

Chapter 33

My Wife's Book Club

In preparation for writing this book, I read several books by writing coaches. They recommend figuring out who your target audience is. My first thought was women, of course; women with disposable income and leisure time. I could see that I would need to pay attention to my wife's book club as one of my target audiences. Fortunately, my wife's book club was planning to invite the husbands to their next book club meeting.

Her book club comprises only women who have the luxury of meeting in the daytime because they don't have jobs. They are not unemployed, as that would imply that they are looking for work. I can assure you that they are not. Most of them had careers in the past but gave them up to raise children. Those children have grown up, and now most of them have children of their own. The husbands of these women have successful careers, so they don't have regular jobs. Some of the women are artists or aspiring artists. Some play tennis, golf, or piano. Some do yoga. Some are docents. Almost all of them do some volunteer work. One of the book club members asked me what I do for volunteer work. I told her that I read to dogs at the public library. That is actually a thing, but I don't do it. That is what I came up with at the spur of the moment as I didn't want to admit that I don't do any volunteer work.

Almost all the members belong to the local country club. My wife and I laugh when we affectionately call them "rich bitches." My wife would also fit into that category, but I could see no benefit in pointing that out. We were both raised without much money, so our mindset is that we will never consider ourselves rich. Even though we are members of the country club, I still buy off-brand canned peaches at the grocery store to save money.

The first thing I noticed about this book club is that it is made up of a very exclusive group of people known as Caucasians. Membership in the book club is somewhat exclusive. You can bring a female guest to the book club, but don't give the guest the false hope that she can become a member because the current membership must approve an invitation to join.

If a club member has a friend who would like to join the book club, the club member is called the nominator, and the friend is called the nominee. The nominator must submit the nominee's name to the chairwoman of the book club for consideration at the next official book club meeting, which is always on the fourth Friday of the month. During those proceedings, the nominator will give testimony or evidence of the nominee's worthiness to become a member. The nominee may be commended based on her ability to continue a conversation while six other women are talking simultaneously. The nominee must be eager to share any rumors or salacious information about the other women in the Green Valley neighborhood and environs. She must do this under the guise of concern so as not to appear to be a gossip. Potential members must be very liberal, or at least appear to be so. If a nominee is wealthy, she is never allowed to admit it. At most, she is allowed to say, "We are comfortable."

The burden of proof of worthiness is on the nominator. A vote is taken. The vote must be unanimous. A ruling is made. There is no appeal.

At least, that is how I imagine how the book club gets new members. All I really know is that membership is exclusive.

Regarding admission to their book club, they never say, "No men allowed," but yeah. No men are allowed.

Once a year, the book club members invite their husbands for an evening meeting. It includes dinner and then a discussion of the book for that month. The dinner is prepared by the host, who must prepare food that fits the book's theme. For example, if the book that month is *Under the Tuscan Sun*, the host would prepare Italian food. I am not a good cook, so if I had to host, I would hope the book would be about Ray Kroc, the founder of McDonald's.

For our upcoming event, they chose a book they thought would appeal to both men and women. It was Bill Bryson's *A Walk in the Woods*. The book is about a very long hike.

The author, and Katz, his friend since his youth, decide to hike the Appalachian Trail. The trail goes from Bryson's home in Hanover, New Hampshire, all the way down the American eastern seaboard to Georgia. They decide to walk it south to north. I would have walked it north to south so that if I gave up on the idea on the first day, I could call my wife to pick me up.

When we got to the book club meeting, we had a nice dinner, and then it was time to talk about the book. I was asked what I thought of the book.

I told them, "As I was reading the book, I pictured a middle-aged, out-of-shape chubby guy, the author, taking his Orson Wells' sidekick, on a 2,000-mile hike. They get through a large portion of the hike when they decide they've had enough. I would have named the book *Two Chubby Smokers Go on a Long Hike*."

I went on, "I enjoy humor, so I was looking forward to reading this book. The book started out funny enough, but then the book started talking about global warming, deforestation, the fragile environment, bureaucrats, botany, and other serious subjects. Possibly the author started out the hike in good humor, but then under the many weeks of hardships on the trail became more introspective and serious." I then added, "I was also a bit disappointed that they didn't finish the hike."

One of the women asked me if I had ever embarked on a long hike. I explained that I had. I had once hiked from Glacier Point in Yosemite to the valley floor.

The woman asked, "Isn't that a hike that is all downhill?"

I replied, "Yes, it is, but I had to take a very exhausting one-hour winding bus ride from the parking lot on the valley floor to the trailhead."

One of the other husbands, Brian, was curious to know if I had read any other Bill Bryson books. I said that I thought I had read most of them. He then asked what my opinion was of Bryson's book, *Notes from a Small Island*, as he was thinking of reading it.

"Well," I said, "I read that book years ago. I believe it was a book about England that Bryson wrote after living there for many years. He tours the countryside and tells us about his adopted country but then appears to run out of cities and sites and starts walking through small villages and onto the beaches."

"I think his book, *In a Sunburned Country*, was similar. He tours Australia, runs out of sites to see, and starts walking in the desert."

Brian then remarked, "It seems that Bryson will write on any subject."

"I agree, he has a book out called: *A Short History of Nearly Everything*."

I then added, "After he wrote the book about everything he was running out of things to write about, so he wrote a book called: *At Home*. He goes through each room of his house and tells you the history of kitchens, halls, hearths, etc. Another Bryson book that brings this point home is his book, *One Summer*. It is about America in 1927. It is about Babe Ruth, Charles Lindbergh, and others. I don't think there is anything in that book that hasn't been written about before.

Brian then says, "Let me get this straight. You don't like Bryson's books, but you have read all of them?"

"I never said I don't like his books. His books don't seem to say that much more than what was already known about a subject, and yet somehow, once I start reading one of his books, I can't put it down. *One Summer* was such an interesting book. If I had read that book when I was in college, I might have become a history major."

I continued my conversation with Brian, "Many of Bryson's books are about walking around. In his book, *Neither Here Nor There*, he takes you on a tour of Europe. Sometimes he walks to a village that doesn't even have a taxi or bus service. It appears to be totally devoid of anything of interest, and yet, in that boring, sleepy town: fascinating and poignant things are happening."

Brian then said, "You know, it just occurred to me that you are good at telling stories about nothing. Some of your stories could be considered neither here nor there." I then told Brian I was actually in the process of writing such a book and was doing research that very evening on what women like to read.

As our book club meeting concluded, the chairwoman asked for book suggestions for the next meeting that would include husbands. I suggested the book *Killing the SS* by Bill O'Reilly, but she said they do not allow the reading of books about war or sports because they are tired of men only choosing from those topics.

She then added, "We also do not accept recommendations from an author from *Fox News* that has paid $13 million to a woman in exchange for keeping her mouth shut about being a victim of his harassment." I responded, "Hmm, your exclusion criteria seem to be rather specific."

The chairwoman then asked, "Did you have any other books that you have read lately that you would recommend?" I responded, "I recently enjoyed a book about Lincoln but that is close to the subject of war."

"I hope you were not going to suggest *Killing Lincoln* by Bill O'Reilly," said the chairwoman.

"Actually, no," I lied, "I was thinking about *Abraham Lincoln: Vampire Hunter*."

Chapter 34

Men Won't Go to the Doctor

Iknew I had to go to the doctor, but I didn't want to. Nobody wants to go to the doctor, but men are more reluctant than women to see a physician. I do not like having my genitals examined by a woman physician or a man physician. I'm sure my patients feel the same way.

I once had to have minor urinary surgery that involved my testicles. I was examined by a U.C. Davis female resident during my preoperative visit. Since she was in training, her physical exam of my genitals was much more thorough than it would have been by the attending physician. We were in a large room when she asked me to drop my pants for her exam. For some reason, the exam room was very large, unlike the small intimate exam rooms I was used to. As I look back on it, it seemed like a gymnasium, and I was concerned someone would walk in on us during the exam. I asked her if I would be given a drape first. She asked if I would like one. I said, "Uh, no." I then asked if a chaperone would be coming into the room. She asked if I would like one. I said, "Uh, no, not really." She then asked, "You are a gynecologist, right?" I said, "Yeah." We both laughed.

I have guilt regarding my reluctance to see a physician when I know I should go. The worst thing a patient can do is to have a serious symptom and then hope it will go away on its own. I have a friend whose father had rectal bleeding. He assumed it would eventually go away and did not tell his doctor until he had symptoms for over a year. He eventually died of colon cancer that may have been cured if found early. The ironic thing is that his son is a gastroenterologist trained at Johns Hopkins. Even knowing this, I postponed my first colonoscopy for eleven years.

Part of the reason men do not feel comfortable accessing healthcare in the United States is because of what could be called the feminization of healthcare. We in healthcare know that women make 85% of the family's healthcare decisions, so we market mostly to women. Labor and delivery units in hospitals seldom make money, but they are a great loss leader. If a woman likes the care she received there, she will eventually be back later in life for her colonoscopy, heart catheterization, and orthopedic surgery. Those services do make money. She will bring her children to that hospital and may even be able to cajole her husband into going there when he has chest pain.

I have a friend who is in his late fifties. His younger brother died of a heart attack in his early fifties. He told me that he does not routinely see a doctor. I tried to get my friend to get a simple cholesterol test. I told him I would feel terrible if his cholesterol was high and no one was doing anything about it. Seeing his reluctance, I even offered to pay for the test myself. His wife told me he wouldn't do it, and she was correct. What makes this more puzzling is that he religiously makes certain that his wife keeps her doctors' appointments. Apparently, he wants his wife to live a long and healthy life, but when his time comes, then he is ready to go. I don't often find women to be so dismissive of preventive healthcare.

The décor in many doctor's offices and hospitals is very feminine. The next time you are impatiently sitting in the waiting room, check to see how many men are there. Waiting rooms are mostly made up of women, children, and the elderly. I have a friend who works for the Merchant Marine. He is out at sea for much of the year, but he takes the children to the doctor when he is home. One time, the receptionist asked to see his Medicaid (welfare) card. She assumed that since he was not working in the middle of the day, he must be unemployed. My friend was not happy.

The magazines in the waiting room are almost always women's magazines. Waiting rooms often have *Better Homes and Gardens, Oprah, Elle, Prevention,* or *Vogue.* Where are the men's magazines? I wouldn't expect to find *Guns and Ammo* or *Soldier of Fortune,* but why do we not find *GQ, Esquire, Motor Trend,* or *Men's Fitness*?

Women are taught from an early age that they will be receiving routine preventive care such as Pap smears, mammograms, etc. Young female patients often have a smooth transition from their pediatrician to a family practice or OB/GYN physician. Men are taught that they should seek medical care if they have an erection lasting more than four hours. Some men don't seek out a doctor for routine care until they are in their fifties. Men don't see health care for themselves as preventive care. Men prefer to "wait until something happens." Many men have told me, "Don't fix it if it isn't broken."

We tend to be very paternalistic about women's health care. We are reluctant to refill a woman's birth control pills if we find she is not up-to-date on her Pap smear. I have often wondered what would happen if a man went into a drugstore to purchase condoms and was told he would not receive them until he had his cholesterol checked and a prostate exam. What if you couldn't buy gas for your car without proof of insurance, evidence of proper tire inflation, and a smog check?

Going to the doctor is not very manly. We men like to think that we can solve our own problems. We do not like to show weakness. I had numbness in both pinky fingers. I thought it might be a minor carpel tunnel problem. It turned out to be a serious spinal cord problem, but I couldn't picture James Bond going to the doctor complaining of numbness in his pinky fingers. When I see Sean Connery on the big screen, do I picture myself in the lead role? "Yesh, of coursh."

Chapter 35

Why Is My Left Hand Numb?

I had noticed for several months that my left pinky finger was numb, but now the one next to it was also numb. Since I am an OB/GYN physician, I know little about medical problems other than those dealing with woman's health.

I thought the numbness could be due to leaving my hand on my abdomen when I slept on my back. I assumed my hand received less blood at that slightly higher elevation, so I started letting that hand rest at my side. That didn't help.

I thought numbness in the hand could be the result of a compressed nerve in the wrist, elbow, or shoulder, so I tried massage therapy, chiropractic, better posture, etc., with no relief from the numbness.

Then I remembered something. I had been using my left hand more. My young female OB/GYN partner, Amy, had been encouraging me to use my non-dominant hand. As we were doing more hysterectomies through tiny "Band-Aid" incisions, she noticed my left hand was not nearly as adroit as my dominant right hand, whereas she was ambidextrous.

She asked me to try some exercises. Instead of doing my usual activities at home with my dominant right hand, she wanted me to use my left hand. I asked her for some examples of things I could try. She said to try doing everything with my left hand, such as eating, combing my hair, brushing my teeth, and even opening a lock with a key in the left hand.

I told her there are some things that I always do with my right hand. She said with a serious look, "Like what?" I replied, "Um, well… I like to butter my corn with my right hand." Obviously annoyed, she said, "Of all the things you could mention, why would you bring that up?"

Could it be that the recent overuse of my left hand was the cause of my left-handed numbness? The answer was no. On careful reflection, I realized that although I had good intentions, I still used my dominant hand much more than my left. For instance, it would be absurd for me to start playing tennis with my left hand. You have no choice but to use your right hand to shift gears in your car.

It would turn out that the left-handed numbness was a symptom of a serious medical problem.

Chapter 36

The Doctor Becomes the Patient

Being the patient gives one a totally different perspective compared to being the doctor. I sat nervously on the exam table, waiting for the surgeon. I was considering surgery for herniated discs in my neck. My legs were dangling. I tried to find something to distract myself while waiting. There was a model of a human spine that I could examine and hold. There were even some metal plates screwed into the vertebrae for demonstration purposes. This was increasing my anxiety. I decided to put the spine down.

It took about fifteen minutes before the doctor entered the room. It seemed like a long time. One expects to wait in the waiting room for a long time, but once you are moved to the exam room, you think you must be next and will be seen quickly. I had no idea how annoying it must be for my patients as they wait for me in the exam room.

Dr. Chau walked in, greeted me with a big smile, and shook my hand. He took a seat next to me. This is a technique we physicians use. If the doctor sits down instead of standing, the patient thinks the doctor spent a lot more time with them than we actually did. It gives the appearance that the physician is not rushed. It would work even better if the doctor leaned back, elevated his legs, and then the medical assistant brought in two iced teas.

He first made small talk about where I was from, what I did for a living, etc. This is also a good patient satisfaction technique to try to make a personal connection with the patient. You are less likely to sue your doctor if you think of him as a person with a family, trying to earn a living. This small talk also gives the impression of not being rushed.

Dr. Chau wore a navy blue suit coat over his light blue scrubs. I have seen men wear a sports coat with jeans, but I have never liked that look. Those men look like they had been gardening when they suddenly realized they were due in court. The sport coat over scrubs was also not a great look. One could not show up at a wedding in that outfit. I think he put on the coat to look more formal out of respect for the patient.

Dr. Chau looked like he was only thirty years old, but it is very difficult to tell how old an Asian is. I am in my sixties, and people have guessed that I was anywhere from thirty-five to sixty. Once, when I was forty, I had to show identification to get into a club where alcohol was served. I wanted to ask Dr. Chau how old he was, but I thought that might not be polite.

Instead, I asked him, "How does a Chinese man get a first name like Dean? He told me he was born in the United States, actually right there at U.C. San Francisco (UCSF) in 1969. That was a relief. Now I knew he was older than thirty. I don't mind young nurses (male or female), but I want my surgeon to have some grey hair.

Since I am Japanese, he asked me if I had a Japanese middle name in addition to my first name of Gary. Most Asian Americans that I know have an Asian middle name. I told him my Japanese middle name was "Whattaguy." He got the joke and smiled.

Dr. Chau did a brief neurological exam and history. He told me I could postpone surgery until my symptoms got worse. I liked that, as it told me he was not "knife happy." Most importantly, he told me that a Hirabayashi laminoplasty would take the pressure off my spinal cord. The approach would be through the back of my neck.

This surgery was my destiny! I had wanted the surgery to be done through the back of my neck. Also, a Japanese doctor had invented the surgery for me, or so it seemed.

This was the first neurosurgeon that told me I could have my surgery through the back of my neck instead of having the approach from the front. I had previously seen two other neurosurgeons, but they did not know how to treat me by going through the back of the neck. One neurosurgeon I had seen previously wanted to do the surgery through the anterior (front) approach and wanted to know why I was reluctant. I said, "There are a lot of vital structures at the front of the neck. What if you traumatize the recurrent laryngeal nerve? Then I won't be able to sing well."

The surgeon asked, "Are you a singer?" I said, "Yes, yes I am. I sing in the car and the shower."

Chapter 37

Flying on a Plane Versus Flying on Propofol (anesthetic agent)

I have a dear friend, Dinah, who loves to go to Kauai to vacation, but she has a fear of flying. It would not be practical for her to travel there and back by boat. Dinah is a nurse. She has absolutely no fear of driving a car but feels that if her car stalls due to engine trouble, she can safely pull over to the side of the road and get help. She feels if the same thing happens on a plane, the passengers will perish.

I quoted her numerous airline safety statistics, but to no avail.

She asked me if I would give her a prescription for Valium to ease her anxiety. I gave her the prescription. She later reported she took the pill at the airport and had no fear of flying (or anything else) on her flight. She has now used Valium effectively on several trips to Hawaii. I don't know if some of this is due to the placebo effect, but what does it matter as long as it works?

According to Dr. Arnold Barnett of M.I.T., if you flew daily on a commercial U.S. flight, it would take you nineteen thousand years before you would succumb to a fatal accident. The same author found that we are nineteen times less likely to die in a plane than in a car, no matter how many times we fly.

When my wife and I drop off our daughter at the airport, we have her call us when she lands to let us know that she landed safely. When she lands, she should actually be calling us to be certain we arrived home without getting in a car accident.

My wife fears flying, although she is willing to fly, anyway. On one trip to Honolulu, as we were landing, she prepared, as she always does for a landing. She looked straight ahead and stiffened her body. She put her head all the way back on the headrest and grabbed both armrests so firmly that I thought she was going to pull them off. I tried to ease her tension by making a joke. I whispered in her ear, "I hope we don't go up in a fireball."

As the pilot was about to touchdown, he suddenly accelerated, and the plane took off into the sky again. I started to panic. What was happening? The pilot came on the intercom and said he saw debris on the runway and decided to make another pass before landing the plane.

On a different trip, my family and I were returning to San Francisco from Honolulu. I was very pleased with myself because I had saved considerable money by booking our trip through a company called SunTrips that offered low-cost charter vacations. I had heard that they used older planes, but I was certain that would not be a problem. We had only been in the air ten minutes when I heard a loud pop. We immediately lost altitude. My daughter told me to look out the window. She asked,

"What is that coming out of the wing?" I said, "That is jet fuel. The pilot is dumping fuel."

The pilot turned the plane around and headed back to Honolulu. I told myself that if we lived through this, I would never book through a discount company again. How dare I put my family at risk just to save a few hundred dollars?

It seemed like an eternity before the captain came on the intercom and told us that one of the engines had failed and we were returning to Honolulu.

When we landed, I thanked the captain for the safe landing and asked him if it was difficult to land the plane with one engine not working. He said, "It was no big deal. I've done it many times before—in the simulator."

For those who fear flying, it really doesn't help to hear terms such as "terminal" and "final approach."

I agree with Dinah. Air safety statistics all sound reassuring until you hit turbulence in your airplane, or you read about a plane accident in the newspaper.

We irrationally think that if we drive a car, we can always take evasive maneuvers and save the day.

I have a friend who doesn't like to wear his seat belt when driving his old truck. He said that he would hope to be thrown clear and land in something soft if he were in a serious accident. I said, "You mean like a haystack?" He said, "Yeah, like a haystack." I replied, "You do realize we live in California and not in Iowa, right? Since you don't drive a convertible, your best hope would be to fly through the windshield and then aim for a car carrying a mattress on the roof."

My friends asked me if I was nervous about having surgery and being put to sleep. I told them that I was comfortable with my chosen doctor and general anesthesia, but was I?

I would let almost any general surgeon take out my gallbladder or appendix, but how does one go about choosing the best doctor for a more complicated surgery? I know how to find a good refrigerator. I go to *Consumer Reports* and check their ratings, but is there a credible organization out there that rates doctors based on specialty? There is an organization called Leapfrog that gives hospitals a safety grade. (I was surprised to find there are hospitals that receive an F.) However, this organization does not rate individual doctors. CMS Compare allows you to analyze physicians in regard to where they trained, etc. but I have known doctors that trained at prestigious American universities and medical centers that were only marginally competent when it came to surgery. Some doctors are excellent when it comes to memorizing or thinking abstractly, but a surgeon has to have manual skills. A lot of that can be learned, but one has to have some basic talent for surgery.

One can quickly find a rating system that evaluates restaurants, but it is not so easy to find a good physician. The evaluations are subjective. Some of the most popular physicians are actually not excellent physicians. I have known surgeons that have no bedside manner; that is, they are abrupt and not empathetic and thus receive poor grades when rated online. Some of these same surgeons have excellent surgical skills.

I remember reading airline magazines that list *The Best Plastic Surgeons in America*, *The Best Orthopedic Surgeons in America*, and *The Top Doctors in America*. Those lists appeared suspect to me, as they looked more like glossy advertisements than the results of a survey. There also seemed to be an overrepresentation of doctors from tourist destinations such as New York and Florida. However, I do like looking at the medical center rating system in *U.S. News and World Report*.

I was surprised to find the email addresses of the heads of medical departments at leading university hospitals can often be found online. Their work email addresses are readily available. I emailed the chairman of neurosurgery at a well-known medical center, and he responded the same day. I described the herniated disk in my neck and asked him who he would go to if he had my problem. He was more than pleased to give me the email address of the doctor he recommended. Of course, it was a doctor in his department, but that didn't bother me. UCSF has an excellent reputation.

One does not have to go to a big-name hospital to receive excellent care. There are world-class doctors in smaller facilities that have honed their skills in one area over many years and have become experts in their field. To me, one of the big advantages of these smaller places is that you don't have residents in training working on you (although residents are well supervised by their attending physicians). Two facilities that come to mind are John Muir Medical Center in Walnut Creek, California, and El Camino Hospital in Mountain View, California. I have no affiliation with either but have considered both of these hospitals for my own cardiac care.

I was very comfortable with my choice of doctor and medical facility, but a lot of thoughts went through my mind the night before surgery. "What if I don't wake up in time and show up too late for the scheduled surgery? What if I wake up in time but the traffic into San Francisco is very heavy and I am so late that they cancel my surgery? What if the chief surgeon allows the resident in training to do the surgery and she makes a mistake? What if I wake up a paraplegic? What if I pass gas in the middle of the case? What if ...."

"What if you stop acting crazy and start thinking rationally like you usually do?" I told myself.

I don't know why but patients often fear the anesthetic more than they do the surgery. Some have expressed to me the fear that they may not wake up. This fear is much greater in those that have never had a general anesthetic.

Although the risk from anesthesia is greater than the risk of flying, it is still very safe. According to the Anesthesia Patient Safety Foundation, there is one preventable anesthetic mortality per one hundred thousand cases. (Hour for hour, the risk of death from anesthesia is about one hundred times that of flying.)

I try to be very reassuring as I stand by the patient as she is about to receive a general anesthetic. Unfortunately, I once made the mistake of saying something that was not reassuring. A patient of mine was being put to sleep for a hysterectomy. I noticed that the anesthesiologist was injecting a white milky fluid into the patient's I.V.

I immediately recognized it as an anesthetic named propofol and I said, "That's the medication Michael Jackson used to go to sleep at night."

The anesthesiologist gave me a dirty look, and I immediately realized my mistake. He was saying, by glaring at me, that I should not be mentioning the anesthetic that Michael Jackson was using as a sleeping aid as the overdose of propofol killed him. It is amazing how much can be communicated by one look from the anesthesiologist.

There are times in our life when we must put our faith in the hands of others. Whether one has to face the fear of flying or surgery with general anesthesia, the best you can do is to consider logic and statistics. Do not dwell on emotions.

When the plane hits turbulence, I now recall that a full 727 jet would have to crash daily, with no survivors, to equal car accidents in the U.S. I recall that on a single flight, the chances of me dying is one one-hundred-thousandth of one percent.

When I am about to undergo anesthesia, I remind myself that the little pulse oximeter on my finger will immediately alert the anesthesiologist if my oxygen level drops so she can quickly intervene. I also remember that I have never seen a patient die from anesthesia.

Chapter 38

Cervical Spine Surgery Day

The UCSF Parnassus campus is very compact. I had been to the underground parking, professional offices, and pre-op areas before the day of my surgery. I now found that the surgical hospital was on the very same block. At my Alma Mater, Loma Linda University Medical Center, everything was more spread out. Apparently, real estate is more of a premium in San Francisco than in the San Bernardino desert.

At my pre-op visit, I had been asked by the nurse and the surgeon if I was taking any ibuprofen. I replied no. It is very important to healthcare professionals that you stop taking ibuprofen before surgery or there could be some excess bleeding. Many surgeons, however, place you on ibuprofen as soon as the surgery is over—when you are still at risk for excessive bleeding—hmm.

I was very nervous but tried not to show it. Everyone in the pre-op area was amicable and tried to make me feel comfortable. I had an anesthesia resident. He asked me if I was on any aspirin or ibuprofen. The Chief of Anesthesia came by and reassured me that even though his trainee would be putting me to sleep, he would be there for the intubation—that is, the insertion of my breathing tube. He also gave me his e-mail address. I told him I doubted that I would be emailing him, but thanked him, anyway. It was a very nice gesture. I thought to myself, "If things go well, I won't need to email him. If things don't go well, I won't be able to email him."

I told the nurses I did not want to receive sedatives in the pre-op area for this surgery. In 2006, I had a minor urological procedure and received a sedative in the pre-op holding area. I didn't remember anything after that and embarrassed myself while under the influence of my pre-op drugs. As they wheeled me to the operating room (O.R.) for the procedure, I reportedly sat up on my gurney and greeted the staff. Of course, I knew them all. My case started at 08:00. My physician colleagues were arriving to start their own cases. They were surprised to see me in a patient gown headed to the O.R. They were concerned and asked me what procedure I was about to have. I told them I was about to be operated on by the urologist Dr. Levine. I told them I wanted my penis to look exactly like his, so I was about to have a penile reduction. I then asked the staff if they could tell me the worst part of having a "threesome." They played along and said they didn't know. I told them that, "When it is all over, the biggest problem is getting all three to agree on pizza toppings." I don't remember saying any of this, but I don't think the staff would go to the trouble to make up such a story.

I was now about to have cervical spine surgery. I told the anesthesiologist I wanted to go into the operating room with my eyes wide open, terrorized like any other patient without any pre-op drugs. I remember being wheeled down the hall into the operating room. That ride down the hall was very short but scary. My wife and confidant of many years, Kathy, was no longer by my side. I remember thinking I was being wheeled down the corridor by very competent people. I was aware of everything around me. I thought, "There is no turning back now."

I remember being told the anesthetic would burn as it entered my vein, but actually, it didn't, and I fell asleep.

Chapter 39

Recovery Room

I awoke to the voice of a nurse saying softly, "Dr. Matsumura, you are in the recovery room now." I remember thinking, "Wow, she knows I'm a doctor. Maybe I will receive special treatment." I then breathed a sigh of relief, knowing the surgery was over. I did not feel as though I had just been put to sleep. I was quite coherent and aware of all that was happening around me, but I knew that I might not remember any of this later.

After I have performed surgery, I speak to patients in the recovery room if they appear wide awake. We have a conversation about how the surgery went. Sometimes the patient will even make a joke. We may discuss a few things, such as the findings at surgery, post-op pain management, and follow-up. Later, the patient will often tell me they didn't remember seeing me at all after their surgery.

My surgery lasted about three hours. After I awoke in the recovery room, I was kept there from 2 pm until midnight because there was no hospital bed available for me.

My wife, Kathy, later told me there was little privacy in the waiting area. Dr. Chau spoke with her immediately after my surgery to let her know all was well. Those seated around her gave a sigh of relief. Kathy was able to listen in on other patients' outcomes. She learned that a lot of them had very rare tumors. One girl from Stockton had just been discovered to have a rare tumor of her scapula the week before. She said I was the only one who appeared to be having "routine surgery."

Once or twice an hour, I would push a button that would immediately give me a dose of narcotic into my intravenous line. When asked by the nurse, I rated my pain three on a scale of one to ten. I was surprised that my pain was not more intense. I did not want to exaggerate my pain level. I find it annoying when I have a patient in early labor that says her pain is ten out of ten as she is smiling and texting on her smartphone.

I often take my wife for granted, but you really appreciate having a loved one around when you feel vulnerable. Kathy asked me if I wanted anything. I said I would really like something to eat. The kitchen had closed, but Kathy had saved a piece of her turkey sandwich that she had eaten earlier. My nurse had been very attentive in keeping me comfortable. I asked her if it was alright for me to eat a piece of a turkey sandwich. She told me that it would be fine, but she was confused as she thought I was a vegetarian. I may have been under the influence of narcotics as I told her, "I am, but I am not a strict vegetarian. For instance, my religion does not allow the eating of bacon, but if I had to choose between eating bacon and going to heaven, it would be a tough decision."

I ate the sandwich and felt much better. I was amazed at how much small favors and kindness are appreciated when you are helpless.

Chapter 40

Foley Catheter

A Foley catheter is a tube placed in the bladder to keep the bladder empty. The other end of the catheter empties into a bag that collects the urine. I have placed hundreds, possibly thousands, of catheters in women's bladders prior to cesarean sections, hysterectomies, etc., and had not thought much about it until my own surgery.

Placing a catheter in a male is a little different from placing it in a female. I don't recall ever having to place one in a male. In a male, you know that the opening (urethral meatus) leading to the bladder is going to be at the end of the penis. In a woman, the opening can be difficult to find, but once you find it, it is easy to thread the catheter into the bladder.

You know you've reached the bladder when you see urine filling the tubing. A balloon is then blown up at the end of the tubing in the bladder so that the catheter will not fall out until the balloon is deflated. The advantage of a catheter is that your bladder will not fill up if, for any reason, you cannot get up to urinate. In my case, I would not be able to walk to a restroom during my time in the operating and recovery rooms.

I can now tell you that it is much better to be the "catheterizer" than the "catheteree." The nurse described how she would be placing the catheter into my bladder and proceeded to do a good job. When she finished inserting my catheter, she asked me what I thought of the procedure. I was very anxious, as I was not sure what to expect. I tried to diffuse the tension by making a joke. I said, "It went well, but you didn't blow up the balloon the way I thought you would."

I had IV fluids running in all day, which causes one to make a lot of urine, so it was nice having a catheter. I thought this would be nice to have when you are on the internet for a long time or are watching a long movie. Alas, I had no idea what I was talking about. I did not know that removing the catheter was going to be painful.

To remove the catheter, the balloon is deflated, and I thought it would then be as painless as removing an earring. It was quite uncomfortable to have the catheter removed, but the worst part was yet to come. For the next twenty-four hours, after removing the Foley catheter, my bladder had painful contractions when I would urinate. My flow would come in seven waves that I could feel. Urinating would make me cry out in pain. I felt as though I was urinating splinters of glass.

Once the catheter was out, I was instructed to urinate into a male urinal that looked like a plastic pitcher. The doctor wanted to measure how much urine I was making per shift. The nurse told me to use it at the bedside, which would save me a trip to the restroom. The first time I used it, I was standing at the bedside, and the food service lady walked in with my breakfast tray. She didn't think this was unusual to walk in while I was urinating, but I found it unnerving.

I immediately walked over to the nurse's station and gave the nurse the order that the measuring of the urinary output had just been discontinued. The nurse informed me that even though I was a doctor, I had no privileges to give orders at UCSF. I told her to call the resident and ask him for a verbal order. I was sure that he would agree with my order, and he did. From then on, I just urinated into the toilet. I soon discovered that if I urinated while sitting down, I was more comfortable and would scream less. I was also able to empty more completely. For the next two days, I found that I would still urinate air bubbles for ten seconds when my urine flow stopped. I'm guessing that was normal.

I think my experience with the catheter was unusual. In some ways, the catheter caused more pain than the surgery. In retrospect, I am grateful to have gone through the experience because it has given me more empathy for my patients. When my patients have pain after their catheter is removed, I will no longer ignore them. Now, I will offer them medication that will numb up their bladder so they won't have to suffer.

By being a patient at the end of my career, I have learned to be more empathetic to the patient, but wouldn't it have been more valuable to have learned this at the beginning of my career? It makes me wonder if medical students should volunteer to have an elective appendectomy as part of their training. They could then learn first-hand what it is like to have to wait in the waiting room, deal with insurance overbilling, be examined by a trainee, receive an intravenous line followed by anesthesia, deal with post-op pain, and the Foley catheter.

Chapter 41

Post-Op Day 1

I was fortunate enough to be given a private room after my surgery. I am guessing that I received a private room as a courtesy for being a doctor. We physicians try to be egalitarian and treat everyone the same, but I know that when I treat a doctor or a nurse, it makes me a bit nervous. When a doctor or a nurse chooses me for their care, it is always an honor and a privilege. I want to be extra careful not to make a mistake, but since we physicians rarely make a mistake, in the back of my mind I wonder if being extra careful to not make a mistake inevitably leads to mistakes. It is best to treat everyone the same and not vary from protocol.

Having been a patient numerous times, I can tell you that almost always the staff knows that I am a doctor and they are particularly nice to me as I am a member of our healthcare family. It doesn't matter that I have never met them before.

The downside to being in healthcare is that the staff thinks that you know more than you do about your medical condition. Actually, we only know about our own specialty. I think the doctors and nurses skip over the discussion of some of the side effects of treatments because they think we have done the research and know the side effects already. I don't think the loss of hearing that I developed after chemotherapy was explained to me clearly. For some reason, I thought all of my hearing would come back. It did not. Possibly, I was so overwhelmed with the diagnosis of cancer that I was distracted and not paying close attention. Ultimately, the permanent loss of some hearing made no difference, as I would have accepted the chemotherapy, anyway.

It is easy to be distracted and not comprehend everything when you are the patient. In my obstetrical practice, I remember the patients always looking forward to having their first ultrasound in the office. Seeing your child's heartbeat for the first time is a magical experience. It makes the pregnancy real. It is also a relief to the doctor when he sees a healthy-looking pregnancy as opposed to a miscarriage or a tubal pregnancy.

On occasion, one sees twins for the first time on that initial ultrasound. I would show the mother the screen and let her make her own diagnosis. I would say, "Here is one baby, and what do you think this is?" I learned early on that once she saw that she had twins, she was in so much shock that she would not remember anything else I would say to her that day. Mostly, she couldn't wait to tell her partner. If I discussed the increased risks that a twin pregnancy involves, such as premature labor and delivery, the extra ultrasounds she would need, or the increased chance of a cesarean, she would not remember any of the discussion. I found that it was better to just let the twin situation sink in and continue the discussion at the next visit.

As I lay there in the dark on my first night after surgery, I became very introspective. I had hoped to go home the day after my surgery. Going home early would save money and since I was a physician, I could probably take care of myself. It turned out that I was not in any shape to do that yet. As I had just had neck surgery, I could barely lift my head.

I became tangled in all the tubes that were inserted into my body. I had two IVs, one in each arm. I had a thin easily tangled narcotic tube that was plugged into one of my IVs. The wheels on my IV pole kept running over that line. There was a small plastic bag of fluid with antibiotics running into one of my IVs. I had a Foley catheter coming out of my penis.

I also had my legs wrapped. The plastic device around my legs would inflate periodically to keep me from getting blood clots in my legs. At my bedside was a telephone line, a nurse call button cord, and a cord to actuate my narcotic dosing machine. All these wires and tubes started to drive me crazy. I felt like a fly caught in a spider's web.

I had just slept from 7:00 p.m. to 2:00 a.m. There was no chance that I would fall asleep now. I needed something to do, but I didn't feel like watching the television.

Despite all these lines attached to me, I decided that I needed a shower. Women may not understand this, but there is nothing worse than having your sticky scrotum stick to your thigh. There was no order in my chart that allowed me to shower yet. There were still concerns that

I could fall. Also, I was not going to have the nurse wake up my doctor to ask him if I could shower.

I decided I was alert and stable enough to shower without a doctor's order as long as I didn't get caught. I called the nurse and told her that I was feeling fine and would like to not be disturbed for a few hours while I rested. I knew it would be a challenge and would take a long time to figure out how to shower with all those tubes attached, but I had nothing better to do. The most difficult part was getting my gown off while keeping the tubes attached to my body. I don't know why I became obsessed with taking a shower. Possibly, the narcotics were not allowing me to think clearly.

I managed to take a shower with two IV poles and a urinary catheter bag hanging out the shower door. When I was done, I found some towels to wipe up the floor. No one was the wiser, and I felt much better.

Chapter 42

Clear Liquids

Warning: I wrote this chapter while under the influence of narcotics.

On postoperative day one, I was given a clear liquid diet. When I saw the clear broth, apple juice, and Jell-O, I knew I would have to say something. I couldn't see any reason why I should not be on a regular diet. I immediately went out into the hall to look for the neurosurgery resident—Dr. Matt, to see if he would order me a regular diet, starting with my next meal.

Doctors often think they know everything and can thus be terrible patients. When I am in the operating room or the delivery room, I am the captain of the ship. It doesn't matter if the patient has uncontrolled bleeding or if her unborn baby is in distress. I am the person responsible, and everyone looks to me to control the situation.

If I make an error or forget something, the staff will make gentle suggestions. I remember once walking into a room where a pregnant patient of mine had just arrived. Her blood pressure was very high, and she was having a seizure. I froze and just stared at the patient for a moment, not believing what I was seeing. The nurse woke me out of my stupor and said, "Dr. Matsumura, do you want to give her something for her blood pressure and magnesium sulfate?" I immediately realized that I was in charge, thanked the nurse for her suggestions, and took control of the situation as I had countless times before.

Well, I don't want to be the doctor that thinks he knows everything when he is the patient and not the doctor in charge. With this in mind, I carefully suggested to the resident that I could probably have my diet advanced to a regular diet. He pleasantly agreed.

I would like to say something about the clear liquid diet. When you have had almost nothing to eat in 36 hours, that orange Jell-O is the best orange Jell-O in the world. You wonder why you don't have it every night, or at least on your birthday. You savor every spoonful as you let the pure, one hundred percent, unadulterated, artificial orange flavor swirl in your mouth for a few seconds before swallowing. Each bite is like eating a spoonful of juicy fruit, without the fruit.

I thought about the chef in the hospital kitchen trying to come up with good Jell-O recipes for his patients that are restricted to clear liquids. The chef could cut an orange in half, squeeze out the juice then add the juice back into the Jell-O powder instead of just adding water. He could then replace the still liquid Jell-O back into the hollowed-out orange halves and serve chilled. What a treat for the patients. If he had a really hungry patient, he could use red watermelon Jell-O in watermelon halves. Mini chocolate chips could be used for the seeds. Why has no one ever thought of this before?

How about pineapple Jell-O in real dugout pineapples? Maybe that is how they serve Jell-O in Beverly Hills hospitals. That's the way they serve Pina Coladas in Maui—in real, hollowed-out pineapples. As I recall, in Maui, those drinks cost a lot! They may have charged us extra because we were tourists. But how would they know we were tourists? Possibly my aloha shirt and my wife's matching muumuu from *Hilo Hatties* tipped them off.

All of these thoughts entered my mind as I ate my clear liquid diet. The clear liquid diet came with a low sodium, low fat, clear broth, which was actually quite tasty. I must get their recipe.

Chapter 43

Sarafem (Prozac)

I have a patient who used to get very irritable before her period. She said she had tension, anger, and irritability for ten days prior to her period. She looked up her symptoms and came up with the diagnosis of PMDD. She was seeing me for a second opinion—her first opinion came from Google.

She said she went to the movies with her husband and some young men were talking too loudly at the front of the theater, so she told them to "Shut the f**k up!" She said it with such authority that they immediately became silent. At that point, her husband gave a (very quiet) sigh of relief. For a moment, he thought the young men might come back to his seat and beat him.

She also found in the days before her period, she would become so emotionally labile that it was interfering with her relationship with her children and husband. She would get very angry with her husband over nothing. He would then say, "Is it your time of the month again?" Actually, it was, but to have him point that out only made her angrier.

She had read about a medication called *Sarafem* in a woman's magazine and asked if I would prescribe it.

I really don't like it when patients badger me for a medication because of direct-to-consumer marketing by pharmaceutical companies. Do the pharmaceutical companies really think I'm going to give a patient their drug just because the patient is going to harass me if I don't give it to her? Does the pharmaceutical company think they can put the drug Prozac in a pretty pastel capsule, rename it *Sarafem,* and then assume I'm going to prescribe it to patients that ask for it by name? All right, I did give it to her. She did come up with the correct diagnosis, and besides, she might be dangerous. I also have to consider this patient may receive a survey in the mail that asks how satisfied she was with her visit with me. A small amount of my pay is based on my patients' satisfaction scores. I gave her the prescription and now we are both happy. Does that make me a sellout? Of course, it does.

Yes, *Sarafem* is simply fluoxetine, which is the generic name for Prozac, but *Sarafem* doesn't have the stigma of the name Prozac, which has become a household name. I think they got the name from the word seraphim, which means angel.

I called in a prescription for *Sarafem* for my patient. When she went to pick it up at the pharmacy, she was denied the medication. Her insurance did not cover it.

It turns out that the pharmacist mistakenly thought I had prescribed *Serophene,* which sounds very similar to *Sarafem. Serophene,* also sold under the name *Clomid,* is an infertility drug not covered by some insurance companies. The pharmacist and I discussed the error, and the patient received her *Sarafem*. Well, actually she received generic fluoxetine, but she was pleased.

This may be one of the few times that an insurance denial benefited the patient.

Chapter 44

Dr. King

I have a good friend, Dr. King. When he was practicing obstetrics, I think he weighed about 350 pounds. He weighs less today, although one would not consider him to be thin.

When Dr. King was waiting for a woman to deliver (which may take many hours), he would sometimes pass the time by cleaning his ears with a paperclip. He would manage to pull out larger amounts of earwax than you would think possible and then form the wax into shapes. Watching him was like driving up to an auto accident—you wanted to turn away, but you couldn't. Once, he molded a small Mallard duck out of the wax, but I thought it looked more like a seagull.

Despite his obesity, he feels he is an attractive man. The surprising thing is that women line up to go out with him. Perhaps they find him attractive because he is a doctor. I don't think it's that simple—there are several single doctors on staff that women are definitely not interested in. One nurse seriously told me about Dr. King, "He is the finest specimen of a man I have ever seen." I think she was blinded by love—he does have an interesting personality and a gentle voice.

One nurse asked him if he would consider dating her. He responded, "I generally only go out with attractive women, but I'll make an exception and put you on my list. My list is pretty long right now and you will have to start at the bottom." She was willing to wait. Maybe the attraction is his brutal honesty.

Dr. King tended to perspire while performing surgery. He would wear a women's menstrual pad—also called a peri-pad—to catch the beads of perspiration from his forehead. A new nurse told me she was shocked when he introduced himself to her wearing a Kotex pad on his forehead.

He and I used to attend an annual OB meeting in Hawaii put on by U.C. Irvine called *Controversies in OB/GYN*. The speakers were excellent. The meetings went from 7:30 a.m. to noon. We wore our flip-flops to the meeting. If the speaker went one minute past noon, he had no audience with us because we were at the Mauna Kea Beach Hotel where the beach was waiting.

Dr. King would wear a Speedo—a tiny swimsuit for men. Most of the swimsuit was covered by his overhanging rolls, so he looked like he wasn't wearing anything at all. I thought if the elastic on his suit broke, it would kill several vacationers.

Dr. King could often be seen riding his Yamaha motorcycle around town. He was easy to recognize as he always wore his light blue scrubs and had his bottom hanging out like a plumber. It was quite a sight to see. He had a large body, yet his feet were small. He wore a size 8 shoe. He laughingly admitted that his motorcycle looked like a moped when he was on it. He once asked me, "Gary, how are a moped and a fat woman alike?" I responded, "I don't know."

"They're both fun to ride until your friends see you."

Once Dr. King and I decided to fly up to Boise, Idaho, to see our retired anesthetist friend, Joe. Dr. King can only walk with two canes due to hip problems. He could not use Joe's shower as it did not have the supporting bars on the walls that Dr. King had installed in his own home. I offered to give Dr. King a sponge bath. This was going fine until I had to clean his genitals. It turns out that the more you clean the genitals, the more there is to clean.

One time Dr. King had an indigent teenage pregnant patient who came in screaming in pain. She had not received any prenatal care. She received an epidural, which gave her immediate relief from her pain. Although still in labor, she was comfortable enough to take a nap. Dr. King asked the pregnant teen's supportive girlfriend if the patient was feeling better. The friend responded, "She's in Seven-Eleven." Dr. King laughed for a week.

Dr. King has a great sense of humor and a heart of gold. It is easy to see why women are attracted to him.

Chapter 45

Body Fluids

Amniotic Fluid

I have an OB colleague who once accidentally drank amniotic fluid. Her name is Dr. Zaidi. When the labor nurse told me this story, I thought she was kidding, but she was very serious. Dr. Z was about to do a delivery. She was gowned and gloved. She asked for the electric bed holding the patient to be raised. The patient was facing her, but Dr. Z had turned to her right to arrange the instruments on her delivery table.

Meanwhile, the nurse had raised the table too high. Dr. Z is short, and the table was now at Dr. Z's neck level. The patient's bag of water had not yet broken. The patient was pushing, and her bag of water was protruding from her vagina like a water balloon.

Dr. Z, having arranged her table to her satisfaction, now turned to face the patient. As she looked toward the patient, the patient gave a strong push, and her bag of water exploded. The water poured onto Dr. Z's face like a waterfall. Dr. Z accidentally took a gulp. We asked her later what it tasted like. She said with a laugh, "It was very salty." Fortunately, the patient did not have any transmissible diseases.

This story reminded me of an episode of *The Tonight Show with Jay Leno*. Jay had been talking about a Southern California woman who had been given the nickname "Octomom." She gained international attention when she gave birth to the first surviving octuplets in 2009. Jay was talking about what it was like when the "Octomom's" bag of water broke. He then showed a clip from the movie *Titanic* where the ship's halls are flooding, and passengers are being washed away.

Breast Milk

There is a condition in which a woman will make breast milk even though she is not breastfeeding. This condition is called galactorrhea. We first examine such a patient to confirm she is making breast milk. We then ask some questions and do some tests.

One patient had this condition, but I could not express any milk from her nipples for confirmation. She said, "You are just not squeezing hard enough. Let me do it." She started further back behind the nipple and then squeezed much harder than I had. She then proceeded to squirt me in the face. She then exclaimed, "Oh, I am so sorry!"

I replied, "Think nothing of it. Women are willing to squeeze themselves much harder than I do. This happens all the time." Actually, it doesn't.

Pus

There are times when we have to open an abscess (pus pocket) of the vulva in the office. I always put drop cloths on the floor before opening a large abscess. I also wear a cover gown as I once had a bad experience while opening an abscess in the office. The pus shot directly onto my necktie.

In that particular case, I opened the abscess with a single stab with a scalpel. The patient, who had been in severe pain, had instant relief. However, the room was immediately filled with a putrid odor from what we call anaerobic bacteria. The abscess had been under pressure, and the contents of the abscess splattered everywhere. The smell was overwhelming and started to spread out into the hall. A young nursing student was watching the procedure from behind me. She later retold the story to a fellow student in the hallway. I couldn't help but overhear her. When she came to the part about the incredible smell, I couldn't help myself, and I said, "I kind of like that smell." The student telling the story then started to vomit. I should have been more sensitive.

I once had a patient who described a terrible odor coming from her vagina that her boyfriend had been complaining about for a month. I asked if the smell was bad enough for him to stop having sex with her. She replied, "Well, no."

I already had a good idea as to what I was going to find with the vaginal speculum. I discovered a "lost tampon" in her vagina. It had been there for over a month. Fortunately, it had not made her sick.

We figured out how the tampon became lost. The patient had had a very heavy period. After placing one tampon, she later added a second. Later she removed one tampon but had forgotten that she had placed two of them.

The patient, of course, was very embarrassed. I was working with a female medical student that day. After the patient left, the student asked me if she should look for an air freshener. I then told her, "An air freshener here would get as much use as Anne Frank's whoopee cushion." She asked, "What's a whoopee cushion?" I replied, "Never mind."

I told her, "Seriously, the best thing you can do is immediately take the soiled tampon in your glove and invert the glove. Next, you tie a knot in the glove and discard it. I then light matches or better yet get out some peppermint oil."

The student then asked, "Well, what if that doesn't work?" I replied, "Then you have no choice but to burn down the building."

Chapter 46

Travel as Diversion

If you ask people what they would like to do in their lives besides getting an education, a career, marrying, and having a family, many will tell you they would like to travel. Apparently, these are some of the things that make a fulfilling life.

I need to travel as a diversion from the stress of daily life. Many doctors have suffered from "burnout," as have I. When we do, we become depressed and cynical. Travel may not be the ultimate solution, but it can help.

When I was in the fifth grade, we sang a song in choir called "Far Away Places with Strange-Sounding Names." It was written by Joan Whitney and Alex Kramer. The lyrics include:

Far away places with strange-sounding names
Far away over the sea
Those far away places with the strange-sounding names
Are calling, calling me

Going to China or maybe Siam
I want to see for myself
Those far away places I've been reading about
In a book that I took from the shelf

I start getting restless whenever I hear
The whistle of a train
I pray for the day I can get underway
And look for those castles in Spain

I felt the calling of those faraway places. I knew that someday I would travel to those places. I was the eldest of four children in a low-income family, but there was never any doubt in my mind, even as a pre-adolescent, that I would someday be exploring ancient walled cities. Families were larger in the 1950s and 1960s. Back then, air travel to exotic places was only affordable for the wealthy. Many American families back then could only afford to go camping for vacation.

My family had a 1957 Chevy. It was copper-colored. We had no idea that car would become a classic someday. When we would go camping, my father would totally remove the back bench seat and replace it with unrolled sleeping bags so we kids could have a soft surface to sit on. We did not wear seat belts back then. Camping for us kids was an adventure. As adults, my wife and I have only camped once. Nice resorts now spoil us. We don't see the point of sleeping on the ground. My wife now says if she wants to rough it, she will stay at the Holiday Inn.

Many of my colleagues tell me they traveled to Europe during their college years. Some were able to stay for months. Myself, I had to work in the summer to earn money for tuition in the fall. I'm not complaining. Tuition is much higher now.

It would appear that college kids today are just as interested in foreign travel as we were in the 1970s. My children were both students at U.C. Davis. I was always amazed at how many of their classmates majored in International Relations. Many of those students spent a year abroad. Can you imagine spending a year in Rome or Edinburgh? Imagine the things you would learn and experience — things you cannot learn from a textbook. It would be almost impossible to spend a year abroad later in life with family and career responsibilities.

I would often ask my children's classmates what they planned to do with their International Relations degrees. One young woman told me she wasn't certain, but she combined it with a second major in French. Another young woman was combining it with economics and thought it would be great to work in a financial institution in Zurich. A young male student told me he planned to get his degree and then join the C.I.A. These are all very admirable aspirations. One of my son's classmates ended up working for an international hotel chain, but as a doorman. It is amazing that when you are young, you can embark on a path of interest without much concern whether it will lead to gainful employment.

In some ways, I am jealous that these students at large universities have so many options. When I was a naïve undergrad at Loma Linda University, a Christian college, I thought my only options were to become a doctor, teacher, or minister. We didn't have a law school. I didn't know anything about engineering. I thought an engineer drove a train — I'm not kidding. My daughter is a civil engineer, and I still don't really know what she does. I picture her at a desk using mathematical formulas.

I have a partner, Dr. Jay. Every year he travels to Scottsdale, Arizona, in the winter to golf and to Seattle, Washington, in the summer to see his family. If he really wants a change of scenery, he goes to Scottsdale in the summer and Seattle in the winter. I get it. It is nice to go somewhere familiar to you. There are no language barriers. You are in a first-world country if you get sick. You can always get a Caesar salad with dressing on the side. Many people enjoy returning to their summer vacation home every year and have fond memories of such—but where is the adventure in that?

Wherever I go, I always consider what it would be like to live the rest of my life in that place. It doesn't matter if I am visiting Kailua, Oahu, or Amsterdam. It's always a wonderful fantasy to think, "What if…"

I love traveling to ancient places and seeing the wonders of the world. Postcards cannot do these places justice. These places are never as I imagined them to be—not even close. To touch the bricks that were placed in the Pont du Gard near Nimes, France, is an experience I will never forget. That aqueduct bridge is 2000 years old. The water flowed in this aqueduct for six hundred years. The mortar holds the bricks solidly—yet the mortar holding the slate on my porch is crumbling.

To stand in front of the pyramids of Egypt, just as Napoleon and the Romans did before us, is something I must do while I can still walk the earth. One must, of course, see where the crusaders left graffiti on the walls of the Hagia Sofia in Istanbul. That is one of the few places where I feel I am still in the fifteenth century, even after I have left the building. Many years ago, we went on our first and only trip to Istanbul. On leaving the Hagia Sophia mosque, we noticed a vendor selling drinks dispensed from a pack on his back. He only had one cup, so he would rinse the cup between customers. He did this by swishing some of the beverage into the cup and then discarding the fluid on the ground.

There are beautiful bronze horses you can see in Venice. They were made during the fourth century B.C. at the time of Alexander the Great. Nero had them taken to Rome. Constantine then had them moved to Byzantium, which had its name changed to Constantinople and is today called Istanbul. The crusaders moved them to Venice. Napoleon took them to Paris. When Napoleon fell, the horses were returned to their "home" in Venice.

How can anyone not want to see these horses and all the rest that Venice has to offer? Many do not desire to see these things, not just because of a lack of financial resources. Many wouldn't mind seeing these horses if the horses would come to them, but the thought of a long flight with the possibility of layovers, flight delays, jet lag, lost luggage, overpriced taxi drivers preying on tourists, the currency exchange, pickpockets, airport security, television in another language, smokers in restaurants, and traveler's diarrhea, make many hesitate to book the flight. What if you come across a toilet that is just a hole in the ground? Is it all a grand inconvenience or just part of the adventure? It can be either one, depending on your attitude.

It is so much easier to see the wonders of the world from a book or a Rick Steves travel log on Public Television, but it is not the same as going there.

Seeing the beach on television is not the same as going to the beach. I remember taking my son to Hawaii when he was three. My son, Eric, always smiled as a child, but his face absolutely beamed when he saw the beach. He looked at the ocean and then looked back at me as if to say, "How long were you planning to keep this from me?" He has never looked back. Someday he will make Hawaii his home, and so will I—at least, that is the dream.

Eric's son is five years old. Finding himself at home in Millbrae, California after a vacation in Hawaii, he asked, "Why are we here and not in Hawaii?" I am still trying to answer that question.

One time Kathy and I were vacationing in Hawaii. My son's family did not go on that trip, but we decided to "Facetime" our grandson. He immediately realized that we were in Hawaii. He left the phone and ran to put on his shoes, thinking it was time to join us.

I have many posters and pictures from my travels in my patient exam rooms. I particularly like to collect ancient maps of Amsterdam, Venice, and other cities. These maps are prints made from the originals. My retired patients love to look at these while they are waiting. They often comment on how they will someday visit these places. I tell them they need to make plans now because "someday" never comes.

One certainly does not have to have a passport to travel to wonderful places. I live in California, yet almost none of my friends are native Californians. Of those from California, I am always amazed at how many have never been to Yosemite National Park. I have been there about twenty times, and every time I go, I ask myself, "Why did I wait so long between visits?"

If you go after the snow melts, you can go up to Glacier Point. You are never the same person after visiting Glacier Point. Things like alimony, acrimony, getting into medical school, etc., all take their proper perspective while you are up there. Even if you never get into medical school or get that job that you desire, you realize that your whole life is but a nanosecond in geologic time. Your life's stresses will all come back to haunt you when you get back home—but for that moment, you realize that eventually, we are all dust. Not that this will make you feel depressed, but it actually makes you feel grateful that you are alive and can enjoy the moment. When I look out over Glacier Point, I feel like Moses looking out into the Promised Land. It is a moment of great introspection. (I recently viewed the Promised Land as Moses did from Mt. Nebo, Jordan. Today it does not look like the land of milk and honey. It looks like a desert.) I also love to gaze up at Half Dome from Fallen Leaf Lake as the afternoon shadows grow longer. The dome often takes on a golden glow in the late afternoon. Then what better way to finish off the perfect day than with dinner at the Ahwahnee Hotel dining room? It is a dining room built like a spacious hunting lodge. Presidents have dined there.

The first time my wife and I had dinner at the Ahwahnee was in 1977, while I was still in medical school. We obtained a reservation for dinner but did not realize that a coat and tie were required for men to dine there. Who brings a suit when you are going camping? Fortunately, there was a jacket and tie I was allowed to borrow for the duration of the dinner. I chose a lime green jacket in a size 44. My actual size is 38. I apparently looked hideous as the waiter found us a table in the corner.

My wife and I were dining that night with another couple. They were both medical students. Elaine is Japanese, and Dennis is Caucasian. We were on student budgets, and we two couples asked for separate checks. The waiter, of course, assumed Elaine and I were a couple—an honest mistake. We had a wonderful evening. We were squandering our student loan money in a four-star restaurant in the most beautiful valley in the world.

I experienced such extravagance again many years later when my son bought me a coffee on St. Mark's Square in Venice for the equivalent of fourteen US dollars. From the outdoor café on the Square, we viewed the bronze horses on the façade of St. Mark's Basilica while a string quartet played. It was worth every euro.

Chapter 47

Contraception

Birth Control Pills

In my opinion, birth control pills have been given a bum rap. Many assume they cause breast cancer. They do not, although they should not be used by someone who already has breast cancer. Indeed, hormones given for years after menopause can slightly increase the risk of breast cancer, but birth control pills are not used after menopause. Birth control pills actually prevent uterine and ovarian cancer.

It is true that women who are on "the pill" sometimes experience nausea, headaches, breast tenderness, etc., but this doesn't occur much more than in women taking sugar pills. Women often say they will not take the pill because it will cause them to gain weight. Women on the pill are gaining weight, but no more than women who are not on the pill. The problem is that we are all slowly gaining weight, but not because of the pill. The good news is that when we get placed in a rest home at age ninety-four, we will all be skinny again.

There are many non-contraceptive benefits to oral contraceptives. These include making one's periods regular. They also decrease the amount of bleeding and the pain associated with periods. They reduce acne and excessive hair growth. Some women take the pill for these benefits and don't even need birth control.

Often, a patient will say she cannot remember to take a pill daily. I then ask if she brushes her teeth daily. She inevitably says, "Of course!" I then ask her if she sometimes forgets and has to write herself a note to remember to brush her teeth. The answer is always no. I tell her to simply put a rubber band around her pills and put her toothbrush in the rubber band. Suddenly a light goes on, and she gets a big smile.

I had been giving this advice for years when I came across a pretty blond teen who was on the pill but couldn't remember to take them every day. I gave her my usual speech, but when I came to the part where I ask if she brushes her teeth every day, she responded, "No." I thought she must have misunderstood the question, so I asked her again. She said she usually does, but she couldn't remember to brush *every* day. I asked if her boyfriend was alright with that. She replied, "Well, we do it doggy ...."

"Alright, alright, I get the picture," I replied. She decided to go with an intrauterine device.

Vasectomy

Vasectomy is a procedure performed on the male to permanently prevent future pregnancies. Although tubal ligation on a female is a simple in-and-out surgical procedure, vasectomy is even simpler and can be performed in the office. One would think most sterilizations would therefore be performed on men.

A common scenario in my practice is that many men will outright refuse to have a vasectomy. Some men will agree to have the procedure, but somehow it never gets done. Before long, the wife is pregnant again. She has the baby and then insists on having her tubes tied during her hospital stay.

I had a patient whose husband agreed to have a vasectomy. He made an appointment with the urologist for a consultation. He passed out at the consultation—that is, he passed out discussing the vasectomy. His wife went on to have a tubal ligation.

Condoms

I have not purchased condoms, but I am told they come in different sizes and in a variety of colors. I understand you can get them with desensitizing gel to prevent premature ejaculation or with ribs for "her pleasure." I assume they come flavored and are available as vegan-friendly and gluten-free. The flavors of strawberry and chocolate sound appealing, but not tuna. I doubt they come in small, medium, and large. They probably come in large, extra-large, and behemoth.

Many patients tell me they are using condoms "every time" until they get a positive chlamydia or pregnancy test. Then they admit they don't always use them.

For women who don't want to get pregnant for at least a year, a Long-Acting Reversible Contraception (LARC) is the best. These methods include IUDs and implants in the arm. These methods do not require a patient to take something every day. These methods can last for years before needing replacement, but there is a problem—LARC does not protect against sexually transmitted diseases. There is nothing wrong with using a LARC and condoms, but I find if a woman is using a LARC, she will not bother her partner to use a condom.

Only condoms protect against sexually transmitted diseases. More condoms are sold to women than to men. It is an easy decision to make in the light of day, but not always in the heat of the night.

Sometimes patients regret they did not use a condom. I asked one patient why she didn't. She replied, "I didn't know him well enough to ask him to use a condom." Well, that makes sense. You wouldn't want to ask such a personal question of someone you hardly knew. Another patient told me, "He was a vegetarian, so I knew he had to be clean."

Chapter 48

Every Time You Go Away

It has happened to all of us. We hear a song on the radio and soon we fall in love with the music. We sing the lyrics to the song, but it turns out we misheard them. Unless someone hears us singing the wrong words and corrects us, we may never learn of our mistakes.

When my son Eric was eight years old, we lived on a street named Rockville Road. One day I heard him singing, "We built this city on Rockville Road." I corrected him and told him that Jefferson Starship was singing, "We built this city on rock and roll."

When I was in college in December of 1973, my roommate Harley started singing a lyric from a song that was popular at the time. He sang, "It's not for you." I said to him, "Harley, the lyric is, "If not for you." He tried to convince me the song was about Christmas morning, and a kid was opening up a present meant for someone else.

My fellow OB/GYN colleague, Amy, and I once attended a surgery center Christmas party. She was reluctant, but I convinced her to come up with me and sing a karaoke song. I chose the song, "Hey Jude." She was familiar with the song, and we did a respectable job singing as the words came across the screen. After our performance, she told me she had always thought the song was called "Hey Jew."

Chuck Palahniuk, in his book, *Consider This*, talks about a conversation he had once with a Scottish journalist who interviewed him by phone. Their conversation digressed to the music they had liked when they were young. The journalist mentioned a Hall and Oates song that had always haunted him. The song was about a girlfriend who stole food from her boyfriend as he gradually starved to death. Palahniuk didn't recognize the song, so he asked the journalist to sing a few bars. He sang, *Every time you go away, you take a piece of meat with you…*.

That same song came up with a patient I was seeing — Janet. I had delivered three of her children. Over time, I started to see Janet more as a friend than a patient. Despite having some difficulties in her life, she had a great attitude. She was also a kindred spirit in that she and I both have an irreverent sense of humor.

One day she came to see me in my office. Her childbearing days were over, so I asked, "What brings you in today?" She replied, "Oh, I'm just here for my Pap smear. It's my lucky day." Then she got a big smile on her face and said, "Actually, it's *your* lucky day!" We had become familiar friends, but not that familiar, as her face flushed with embarrassment. We then both had a good laugh.

It turned out that her Pap smear was abnormal, so I called her the next day to ask her to make a follow-up visit.

When a woman has an abnormal Pap, she will often need a microscopic exam of her cervix to see if she has cancer or pre-cancer. This is done as an office procedure called a colposcopy. The patient places her feet in stirrups as she lays on her back on the gynecologic table. A speculum is then placed in the vagina. The cervix is visualized at the top of the vagina. A microscope is then positioned to look up the vagina and onto the cervix.

From there, "biting" instruments with jaws are used to take small biopsies from the cervix. These specimens are small, about the size of half a grain of rice. No anesthetic is given, so a small amount of pain is involved. The tiny pieces are then placed in a small vial of preservative fluid and sent to pathology for diagnosis.

Unfortunately, the results came back inconclusive, so Janet had to return and go through the procedure all over again.

This time, Janis asked to look at the pieces of her cervix settling in the bottom of the specimen bottle. She asked, "What happens to the pieces of the cervix once the pathologist is done looking at them?"

I replied, "I think he keeps the pieces and makes a snow globe out of them."

With the specimen bottle in my hand, I was leaving the procedure room to let Janet get dressed when she said to me, "Before you go, I have a song I want to sing to you." I said, "Go ahead."

She sang, *Every time you go away, you take a piece of me with you.*

Janet is one of my favorites—no, she is my favorite patient. Each visit after that one, I would take the opportunity to greet her with, "Is today my lucky day?"

Chapter 49

Thailand and Cambodia

Sometimes I suffer from burnout, especially if I have had some rough call nights. I keep my phone on vibrate, but when sleep deprived, I feel phantom vibrations and think my phone is vibrating when it is not. I have often wondered if I should have gone into dermatology so I could sleep all night undisturbed. Do dermatologists get called for emergencies? What would be a dermatologic emergency? Possibly one would be a teenager getting a pimple just before prom night. I'm sure my dermatologic colleagues would not appreciate that comment.

One of my patients showed up in the Emergency Room at 3 a.m. because the bleeding from her vagina had stopped. She had bled daily for thirty days, but now the bleeding had stopped. She was worried she had run out of blood. That same night, a pregnant patient called to tell me she couldn't sleep. Once in the middle of the night, a pregnant woman called to tell me that she had a toothache. I told her she needed to call her dentist. She exclaimed, "Doctor, do you have any idea how late it is?"

I can better tolerate my busy work schedule if I have a travel adventure on the horizon. One can suffer through any number of sleepless nights if your next trip is to Thailand.

Bangkok Restaurant

When we got to Bangkok, our guide, Dum, referred us to a Thai restaurant near our hotel. It was excellent and dinner for four only cost about $30 U.S. dollars. Dum told us that the Thai people do not consider the food good unless it is very spicy. By spicy, he meant spicy hot. We did not want to eat food that would be too spicy for us to handle, so Dum told us to say, "Mai-pet," and they would know to tone it down.

I asked the waitress if she could substitute tofu for chicken in the red curry dish. The waitress did not speak much English, but she wanted to know if I was a vegetarian. She asked, "Are you a vegetable?" My wife responded, "Yes, he is."

We told the waitress we wanted the food to be "Mai-pet." She gave an understanding smile. Our food came out mild except for the green papaya salad, which was very hot from the ground-up peppers in it. I think they may make the salad in advance. I decided to put out the fire by eating some of my red curry dish. I then bit into a small green bean. Well, I thought it was a green bean, but it was a small pepper. I considered spitting it out for a moment, but then I thought, "It isn't that hot." As the seconds went by, the sensation became more intense. My eyes began to water. Soon, I was not able to focus my eyes. Drinking tea and water was not much help. Relief only came with time.

This reminded me of a party I had attended with fellow physicians years ago. One of the doctors was from the Midwest and thought he was taking a bite of guacamole when it was actually wasabi, a green Japanese horseradish condiment. It is very pungent and burns the sinuses. I use it so sparingly that the amount I put on my sushi is barely visible. The Midwest doctor was in such agony that we thought he was going to have to go to the emergency room.

Bangkok Massage

Massage establishments can be found on almost every block in the tourist shopping areas of Bangkok. Sometimes you can find three on a single block. The legitimate massage businesses are strictly for massage and not sex. The sex trade is there but must work out of other venues. The massage businesses are easy to identify as each establishment has all of their young massage therapists wearing the same color tee shirts. When things are slow, there may be eight massage therapists sitting outside the entrance. Several may approach you, saying, "Massage, you want massage?" When I was there years ago, they charged from $7 per hour. Massages in the hotels were more expensive.

The most expensive massage I obtained was $60 for two hours. It was in a very private and clean establishment that included a shower. I went back to this place for three nights in a row. I couldn't pronounce my massage therapist's name very well, so she asked me to ask for number 75 the next time I came in. She worked seven days a week with three days off per month. She spoke hardly any English. She asked me to shower and gave me some standard-issue massage underwear. The underwear was sheer, disposable, and came packaged in only one size, small. I accidentally tore my underwear, trying to get into it each night. My adult son could not get his on any higher than his knees, so his massage therapist told him to skip it.

I was getting out of my shower when the therapist knocked on the door to see if I was ready. I called out, "I'm not ready yet." In Thai, that must translate into, "Please come in. I'm ready." She came right in and prepared her table as I toweled off.

A Thai massage is a combination of Swedish massage and wrestling. You can expect to be a bit sore after the massage, although not bruised. I would cry out, "Ah, ah!" My therapist would then ask, "You hurt, you hurt?" I did not want to appear unmanly, so I would give out a weak "no." She would then resume with just as much vigor until I cried out again.

At times, the therapist entwines her body with yours and then stretches you out. If someone walked in on your massage, they would think you were fighting. Even when I was young, I could not do the splits, but I could at the end of my Thai massage. In the end, the therapist would have me sit up, as she would do some range of motion exercises on my arms and back. If there was a cracking sound, the therapist would give out an "ah" of approval.

Before my second massage, I decided to give my massage therapist, number 75, a heads up that I wanted her not to do such a deep tissue massage. I remembered what Dum had told me to say at the Thai restaurant, so I said the only Thai phrase I knew, "Mai-pet." I thought that meant "tone it down." Dum later told me that was not an appropriate phrase to use in that situation, as it means, "Not too spicy."

Cambodia

Cambodia is an impoverished country. Our guide there was Khett.

Almost everyone in Cambodia has lost at least one family member to the Khmer Rouge army. Khett's oldest brother was conscripted into the Khmer Rouge army and later killed by the same army as Pol Pot went about killing millions of his own people. Nevertheless, the Cambodians smile a lot and are the gentlest people I have ever met. Many can speak a fair amount of English.

Khett said the average income in Cambodia at that time was less than $700 per year. He bragged that the average income in Cambodia was higher than that in many parts of Africa. I guess you can always find people less fortunate than yourself, even if you have to look on another continent to find them.

Chapter 50

Dr. Pepper

Dr. Pepper is the oldest major soft drink in the United States, according to The Dr. Pepper Museum. Dr. Charles Alderton invented it, a young pharmacist working at Morrison's Old Corner Drug Store in Waco, Texas, in 1885. (Coca-Cola would be introduced the following year.)

The drugstore had a soda fountain. Alderton liked the smells of the drugstore, so he started experimenting with flavors that would reproduce the fruity aromas of the store in a drink.

Alderton offered his new drink to owner Wade Morrison who liked the drink. The soda fountain customers also liked it and called it a "Waco."

Morrison is given credit for naming it Dr. Pepper, but no one is certain about how he came up with the name, although there are many theories. Fortunately, he did not name it after the inventor, or today we would have to say, "I'd like to order a large Dr. Alderton."

In the 1920s and 1930s, a typical country doctor character with a monocle and top hat became the Dr. Pepper symbol for the company.

In the 1920s, Dr. Walter Eddy at Columbia University was studying human metabolism. He found that people had a natural decrease in energy at about 10:30 AM, 2:30 PM, and 4:30 PM. He also found that if one had something to eat or drink at 10, 2, and 4, the energy slump could be avoided.

The Dr. Pepper advertising agency got busy. They decided that the ingestion of sugar at 10, 2, and 4 would be healthy, and what parents wouldn't want their children to be healthy? They pushed the idea that Dr. Pepper had quick energy sugar the body needed and healthy water. What was there not to like? 10, 2, and 4 would become "Dr. Pepper Time."

The older bottles of Dr. Pepper had the numbers 10-2-4 on the label positioned as they would be on a clock. Those bottles now belong to collectors, but old advertising signs and painted barns in the South still display those numbers.

The beverage tastes a bit like prune juice, but the company says that prune juice is not one of the ingredients. Nevertheless, some believed it should be imbibed at the prescribed hours to prevent constipation.

We physicians often prescribe medications with the directions to the pharmacist written as TID. TID is a Latin abbreviation that means three times a day. One has to wonder if, years ago, people thought that Dr. Pepper was a legitimate medicinal.

My aunt collects baubles. Almost every room in her house is filled with keepsakes. I noticed she had one of the classic glass bottles that had the 10, 2, and 4 logo in her collection.

My aunt and I were watching the news on television when an elderly woman in Fort Worth, Texas, was shown being interviewed. Her name was Elizabeth Sullivan, and she was celebrating her birthday at age 104. She was asked what the secret was to her longevity. She started drinking Dr. Pepper after age sixty. She said, "I started drinking them about forty years ago — three a day."

The interviewer asked the elderly lady what her doctors thought of her drinking Dr. Pepper three times a day. She said, "They told me it would kill me."

"What do they think now?" asked the interviewer.

"They're all dead."

Chapter 51

Refusing a Cesarean

A patient of mine came to the hospital in labor. Soon after her arrival, her doula came in. A doula is a labor coach. She is a non-medical person who assists the patient before, during, and after childbirth. During active labor, she is there to give physical assistance and emotional support to the patient.

The role of a doula is to help the mother feel safe and comfortable. The goal of the doula should be and generally is the same as that of the doctors and nurses, which is to ensure a safe delivery for mother and baby. Doulas should have no clinical role — that is, they should have no medical decision-making authority, instead, deferring to the nurses and physicians.

The doula provides physical assistance such as giving a massage, assisting the patient with a warm shower or an inflated birthing ball, placing the patient in various supportive positions in the bed, providing liquids or ice chips, etc.

The doula provides emotional support by encouraging the patient through a long and challenging labor. The doula often reassures the patient that the fetal heart rate is normal, reminding her there will be a wonderful reward at the end of the delivery to make the ordeal all worthwhile.

Months before the baby is due, the doula educates the patient about the birthing process. Part of this is to relieve the fear of the unknown and help the mother develop a birth plan. The birth plan allows the patient to take an active role in the birthing process.

Doulas provide support for only one patient throughout the active labor process. On the other hand, nurses and physicians are busy taking care of multiple patients and usually provide intermittent care during labor. Doulas give needed encouragement to patients to persist in their long labors and keep pushing long after the patient would have liked to have quit. Often the patient would have given up and asked for a cesarean section were it not for a very supportive doula.

I want to make it clear that just as most physicians are providing excellent care, so are most doulas providing a valuable service to patients.

It is important to stress that doulas do not have formal medical training. I take issue with a minimal number of them if they choose to give medical advice and direct the patient away from interventions that can be lifesaving. This is often done in the name of natural childbirth. Some doulas will try to steer patients away from receiving pain relief, such as an epidural. Unfortunately, some doulas have a personal agenda. They think modern health care has conspired to make the delivery process unnecessarily impersonal and sterile.

I recall a particular patient who brought a doula with her. The patient had a birth plan, which is common among mothers, especially if it is their first delivery.

After being in labor for a while, the fetus' heart rate started to go down after contractions. The fetus had the most ominous of fetal heart rate decelerations called late decelerations. If these drops in the heart rate do not resolve and the patient does not deliver vaginally within a certain time frame, then at some point, there must be a procedural intervention (cesarean or instrumented vaginal delivery) to prevent permanent harm to the fetus. The mother was informed of this.

The doula informed the patient that childbirth was a natural occurrence and she should not be concerned. The patient was advised to switch to more accurate monitoring of the fetal heart rate so the fetus could be observed more closely. The doula advised the patient this was unnecessary and that internal monitoring of the fetal heart rate by placing an electrode on the fetal scalp could cause damage to the baby. I reassured the patient that placing the monitor on the fetal scalp offered considerable benefit, with almost no risk. Still, the patient decided to follow the advice of the doula.

The fetal heart rate continued to deteriorate. The recommendation to have a cesarean was refused by the patient based on the doula's advice. As the parents would not take my advice, I asked the mother if I could obtain for her a second opinion from another obstetrician who was waiting for one of her patients to deliver. The patient agreed that there would be no harm in obtaining another opinion. The second obstetrician confirmed my assessment. She told my patient that a cesarean was necessary or the consequences to the newborn could be brain damage or death. The second obstetrician was calm and respectful.

The patient asked for a moment to discuss the second opinion with her doula. My patient was convinced that childbirth was a natural process. Nature knew best, and she decided that the birth process should continue without any intervention.

I was frustrated. I explained that childbirth was often uncomplicated and uneventful, yet at other times carried significant risk. Prior to modern medicine, neonatal death was common as was maternal death. I recalled that President Thomas Jefferson's wife Martha had six children, but three died as infants. After delivering her last child, she herself died from complications of childbirth. My patient was firm in her decision. I felt as though I had failed as a physician. How could my patient choose to disregard my professional advice?

Finally, the baby girl delivered spontaneously. The newborn was quickly taken to the warmer, but was blue and not moving. The doula insisted the baby be brought back to the mother to allow immediate breastfeeding, which is the routine if the baby is breathing. She was informed that the baby did not have a heart rate, and resuscitative measures were being given by the neonatologist. Ultimately, the baby did not survive.

Some of the nurses were traumatized by the delivery and were given counseling. The nurses had never watched the fetal heart rate continue to deteriorate before their eyes without intervention. They knew a cesarean could save the baby. The nurses would all go through a debriefing. All were given a chance to offer up suggestions as to how this could be avoided in the future. We developed a doula policy.

Now when a doula is brought in, she must sign a lengthy document that carefully defines her role. If she tries to direct the patient's medical treatment, she will be escorted out by security. We want to be a welcoming unit to all, but our first responsibility is to be an advocate for the patient and her unborn child.

The parents do not need to be punished, in my opinion. They experienced the worst form of punishment a parent can experience — knowing that they refused an intervention that could have prevented harm to their child. In regards to the doula, I'm sure she was well-intentioned. She had wanted this couple to have the best experience possible. Hopefully, she learned a lot from this experience.

I have seen patients, with and without a doula, refuse a cesarean in the face of a life-threatening fetal heart rate, and yet in some of those cases the baby came out just fine. We doctors are not always right. Fetal heart rate monitoring is not an exact science, but wouldn't you rather have someone interpreting the pattern who has monitored thousands of women in labor as opposed to someone who has had no formal training?

I had a couple come to me for prenatal care with concerns about a previous pregnancy. The husband said that in the previous pregnancy, their lay midwife had recommended a home birth. (I do not recommend home births under any circumstances, but I will admit that most of them go well.) During the labor, the wife started to bleed—a lot. She had been told the hospital was an uncomfortable place to have a baby and was full of sick people and germs. She became scared and locked herself in the bathroom. The husband coaxed her out and brought her to the hospital where she underwent an emergency cesarean. The placenta had prematurely separated while she was in labor. That was the cause of the bleeding. Without the placenta attached to the mother, the fetus could not get oxygen. The baby did not survive.

The husband and his wife later divorced. I don't know if it had anything to do with the delivery. The husband remarried. He and his new wife were now coming to me for prenatal care. He said that he had been so traumatized by the previous delivery that they had decided to have a totally elective cesarean in the current pregnancy and not even attempt a vaginal delivery. My heart went out to him. I told him we could discuss that or they could attempt a vaginal birth in the hospital.

Chapter 52

Taking Tennis Too Seriously

Due to the stress in our lives, I think everyone should participate in a regular exercise program. Traditionally, we think of doctors as being golfers. Golfing may be very enjoyable, but to an uninterested spectator like me, it looks rather boring. I have a family practice friend that says he would prefer to give up sex rather than golf. I hope he doesn't tell his wife about this preference. When people ask me if I play golf, I say that I am too thin to play golf. This does not make me very popular with golfers.

I find that I can play tennis for three enjoyable hours. I could never work out in a gym for more than an hour without getting bored.

Nevertheless, tennis can be very frustrating. Many amateur tennis players, including myself, think that they are better players than they really are. Shots that I can handle in practice become much more difficult in a real game. I can handle 90% of my overhead shots when practicing but only 60% in a U.S.T.A. League match.

Tennis matches are not necessarily relaxing. Look at the intensity of the faces of professional players as they play. Although league matches create tension, at least one forgets about all the other problems one has in life while playing. Instead, you focus on the lob that you just sent up that was called "Out!"

I once saw a fellow player throw down his racket and go home after a bad line call. This was during a practice game! We all take amateur league tennis very seriously. I am not sure why. It is not as though we are ever going to be playing in the US Open. I have never won a trophy or even a mug, although I did receive a tee shirt when our team made it to the district playoffs.

One of my good friends is a family practice doctor. He is the most gracious man you could ever hope to meet. He is generous, cordial, and sensitive. However, when he gets on the court, if he starts losing, everything changes. He throws his racket on the ground, makes bad line calls, and starts yelling at himself.

This family doctor loved tennis more than anyone I have known. On a Sunday, he would play in the morning and again in the afternoon. If someone then called to see if he was available to play, he would go out again in the evening. On weekdays, he would play at 6 AM.

This doctor passed away in his mid-sixties. We started a tennis foundation in his name. This foundation sponsors a $100,000 Men's Pro Invitational.

During this tournament week, I was able to play in a Professional-Amateur (Pro-Am) match. I was matched up against a tall, lanky, affable player. I introduced myself as Gary, the team doctor for that night, and welcomed him to the tournament. I asked him to give me his best kick serve to my backhand, as I wanted to see if I could return it. I asked him not to hold back. I was able to make contact with the ball, but I could not keep it within the court.

I later saw that he was serving much harder to some other younger amateurs. I think he realized that he did not want to accidentally injure the old team doctor.

The U.S.T.A. requires that there be a doctor at these professional matches. We now have orthopedic physicians participating in that role. I am not certain how useful I would be if there were an injury at one of these games as an obstetrician/gynecologist. I could call for an ambulance if someone was seriously injured. I would also be comfortable with a spectator going into labor, but that is not likely to happen.

These young professional players are not likely to need a physician on-site to care for a life-threatening injury. It is much more likely that an older spectator, like me, will have a heart attack.

Years ago, tennis was more formal and played with proper etiquette (think Wimbledon). I thank John McEnroe for lowering the bar with his famous rant against the chair umpire that would start with: "You cannot be serious!" It is no longer always a gentleman's game. By reading players' lips, I have noticed a modest amount of foul language in men's and women's professional tennis.

I was once practicing with my friend Dr. Levine at the Rancho Solano courts. We were having a friendly Saturday morning practice, and we were talking a lot between points. The two women playing in the next court became annoyed with our talking. Finally, one of the women spoke up and said, "Would you two please shut up?" My friend responded, "Oh, I recognize you. Your team is called the cunning runts."

My wife and I don't play mixed doubles anymore, at least not with each other. We tried to play together, but it didn't work out. If I was playing with someone else's wife and she made a mistake, I would say, "Good try." When my wife makes a mistake, I may say, "I thought I told you to watch your alley." She then responds with, "I thought I told you to shut up!"

I once played a singles match against a woman from a Vacaville tennis club. She asked me if I had called her last ball out. I replied that I had a perfect angle to see the ball, and it landed just a few feet from me outside the baseline. I told her that I clearly saw the ball as out. She said to me, "In that case, you are a cheater and a f**ker!" I responded, "I'm not a cheater."

Chapter 53

Forgetting Our Ethnic Origins

One of my best friends is a family practice physician. He and his wife are both of Italian ancestry. They both have light brown hair and blue eyes, so I would not have known that they were Italian if it were not for their very ethnic-sounding last names. His first name is Christian. A friend once asked his mother-in-law if her ancestors came from northern or southern Italy. The mother-in-law took considerable offense at this question, became very depressed, and would not come out of her house for a week.

Christian asked her why she found the question so offensive. His mother-in-law replied, "Most of my ancestors are from northern Italy. We consider ourselves Europeans. We consider southern Italians to be more Mediterranean. They are darker. They are often from Naples or Sicily, which are considered Mafia strongholds."

I told Christian I had heard things were similar in Japan, that is, the people in northern Japan considered themselves to be of a higher class than those on the southern island of Okinawa.

Christian knew the woman asking the question had meant no offense and felt no offense should have been taken. He wanted to know what I thought. I said, "I don't think your mother-in-law should have taken offense, but one has to be very sensitive whenever one brings up the subject of race or ethnic origin. I always assume if the topic of race comes up, someone is going to take offense. I always enjoy it when someone starts a sentence with, 'I'm not racist, but have you ever noticed….' That means they are about to say something offensive."

I continued, "I want you to know that I don't care if your ancestors came from northern or southern Italy. You will always be a Dego-Wop-Guinea to me." Christian smiled.

We have another family practice physician in our group who is a good friend of mine. His name is Stephano.

I once said to him, "Stephano, did you know I'm going to Italy this spring?

He replied, "No, what are you going to see?"

I said, "I want to revisit Naples, this time at my leisure. It has Mount Vesuvius, Herculaneum, Pompeii, and the National Museum, where the treasures of Pompeii are stored. In the museum is a separate adult erotic section. Suppose we had a six-foot painting of a penis in our living room. That would be considered to be in poor taste, but in Pompeii two thousand years ago, that was considered art, a celebration of fertility. I heard about this museum when I was in college, but we didn't have time to see it on our escorted tour several years ago.

Stephano: "I heard Naples was a rough town."

Gary: "That is true, but I always felt safe there. Maybe the Mafia keeps the town safe for tourists, so the tourist dollars will keep flowing in. I have heard it is probably better to stay in Sorrento and visit Naples by boat. Have you ever been to Naples?"

Stephano: "I've never been to Europe."

Gary: "Whoa, whoa, whoa. Non si fa cosi! (That's awful!) Your last name, DeNapoli, means 'from Naples,' and you have never been to Italy? Stephano, the greatest tourist destination in the world, is Italy. You should be ashamed of yourself."

Stephano enjoys playing guitar. I play the ukulele and bass so we have done duets for parties. One night we were practicing the song "Somewhere Over the Rainbow." I noticed he was playing so loudly that my little ukulele could hardly be heard. I said, "Stephano, you need to play more softly. You need to play mezzo-piano."

He asked, "What does mezzo-piano mean?"

I replied, "It means softly." I then added, "Do you mean to tell me that your name is Stephano DeNapoli, and you don't speak any Italian?"

He responded, "No, I don't speak Italian. Do you speak Japanese?"

I said, "Oh...."

Chapter 54

Woman Refuses to See a Female Doctor

Many women do not care if they see a male or female obstetrician at their delivery, but some definitely feel more comfortable with a woman. If a woman insists she wants to be seen by a woman physician only, we tell her we can't guarantee that a woman will be available to deliver her as we have male physicians — such as me — in our call group. Although our practice is comprised of mostly female obstetricians, it would not be fair to ask them to be up for an extra night of call to satisfy a patient's preference.

I tell women if it is that important to them, they should switch to a practice made up of all women.

I once had a black woman tell me she preferred to see a male physician. She admitted she had this old stereotypical preference in which she pictured a competent doctor as being male, white, and older. She would not prefer a black or female obstetrician. I said to her, "I noticed you said white. What do you think of me?"

"Oh," she said, "I accept you as an honorary white."

I then said, "Alright, I think that was supposed to be a compliment."

I told her that I did not think she would find a local, all-male obstetrical practice, although it would have been easy to find one forty years ago. She admitted it was a ridiculous preference and said she would accept whoever was available for her delivery.

There have been many occasions in which a woman shows up in labor and informs the nurses that she only wants a female obstetrician to deliver her even though she had never mentioned that preference in any of her prenatal visits. If the patient can be accommodated, we honor the request. If a female obstetrician is not available, I have a strategy that generally works.

I go into the labor room pretending that I don't know the patient's preference for a woman doctor. I make eye contact, shake her hand, introduce myself, sit on the edge of the bed for a moment and briefly discuss her pregnancy. I studied her chart before entering the room, so she soon realizes I have made every effort to make myself aware of any issues in her pregnancy. I go out of my way to accommodate special requests if possible. I ask her if she has any questions, and then I leave the room.

The patient will almost always tell the nurse to disregard her previous request and that she finds me acceptable to deliver her baby. I am five foot, six inches tall, not muscular, and I have a soft voice. Since I am not very manly, I think gender preference becomes less important.

I once had a patient who requested that she *not* be seen by a woman physician. Her name was Marisol, and she was a model. I asked her why she could not see a female. She said that women were often jealous of her body and treated her in a very catty way. She started to tear up as she spoke. I did not ask for details.

I told her I was sorry, but she would have to take her chances, and it was likely that a woman would be on call the night she went into labor. I admit I did not take her very seriously.

One day while I was taking call, the nurses told me Marisol had come in the day before as she thought her bag of water had broken — it had not. The first thing Marisol asked was whether a woman or man was on call. When she learned it was a woman, she started crying. When I heard this, I realized she must have had some traumatic events with women in the past. I decided I would come in special for her when she went into labor. It was not just that I was so sympathetic to her cause — which I was — but also, I was starting to bond with this patient as she had only seen me, and none of my partners, during the entire pregnancy.

It takes quite a commitment to guarantee a patient you will be there for her delivery. It means possibly having to leave a social engagement or cancel a tennis game. I would not be able to plan any vacations near the time she was due. I am rarely willing to make this commitment.

When I told Marisol I would attend her delivery, she was very grateful as she breathed a sigh of relief.

When she became thirty-six weeks pregnant, I asked her if she thought it was still safe for her to be wearing her six-inch high heels. She said she might trip without them because she was so used to wearing them.

When Marisol went into labor, she presented herself to the labor and delivery suite at the hospital. She told the nurse she did not want to be examined by a woman and that Dr. Matsumura had consented to be called even if he was not on call. At first, the nurse thought she had misunderstood the patient. The nurse asked, "Are you sure you only want to be examined by a man? Are you sure Dr. Matsumura said to call him even if he was not on call?"

I came in and did the delivery, which went well.

Marisol was very grateful to me for making her more comfortable in her birthing experience. She decided to give me a gift. Before delivery, she had some tasteful nude pictures taken of herself with her pregnant belly showing. In the photos, she stood to the side with her arm strategically placed. The images were very professional-looking, just as the pictures of Demi Moore were when she posed nude and pregnant for the magazine *Vanity Fair*.

Marisol was very proud of these pictures and gave them to me framed. I displayed them in my office.

Some of the medical assistants thought the pictures were in poor taste. What if some of my other patients saw the pictures and thought I collected photos of naked pregnant women? I quickly took down the pictures and only displayed them in my office when I knew Marisol was to be my next patient.

Chapter 55

Dirty Microwave

We have a microwave at work—as most people do at their place of employment. After a while, it looks and smells like someone gave birth in there—a week ago.

I don't see why I should be the one to clean it. It would take a chisel to get the food off the inner walls and ceiling of that oven as the splattered food has been baked on. It would be like trying to get graffiti off of a wall. I certainly wouldn't mind cleaning up my mess, but this isn't my mess. It would take quite a bit of time to clean and I have to get back to work. This is probably the attitude most people take and the microwave doesn't get cleaned until someone can't take it any longer.

Finally, one of the more assertive nurses—Debbie—will clean it and then leave a scathing note on the door about how inconsiderate we are for not covering our food and cleaning up after ourselves. The messages tend to be quite aggressive as Debbie is probably seething the entire time she is cleaning.

I always assumed women were cleaner than men. Men's public restrooms can be pretty dirty. I remember going to a movie theater restroom once, and on entering a stall, I noticed there was urine on the back wall of the door. A man does not always have good aim when he urinates, but how does one get urine on the wall behind him?

I'm reminded of a story I would like to forget. When I was in medical school, my friends and I used to go to the library at the University of California at Riverside to study at night. We found that we studied much better in a library as it did not have all the distractions of a dormitory. During our breaks, my three friends and I would try to amuse ourselves. One day my roommate gave us a challenge in the form of a bet. He would offer up all the change in his pocket versus all the change in our pockets. The bet was whether or not he could urinate at least one drop of urine over the library's public restroom stall door. That seemed impossible even though he was over six feet tall. My roommate took out his penis and rocked his body back and forth. He then let out a big spray of urine with a hoot, and sure enough, some of it went over the door. We were all laughing hysterically until we realized our pants and shoes were wet.

I assumed it was just men that would leave a mess in the food prep area, but our labor and delivery department is made up of almost all women. I was discussing this with one of the nurses when she told me that the week before, she was in the employee women's toilet stall when she noticed above the toilet tissue dispenser someone had placed her sanitary pad that had been soaked with blood. Apparently, the employee was disgusted with her situation at that moment and slammed it onto the stall's wall where it stuck. The point is — not all women clean up after themselves.

I immediately saw this as an opportunity to spread the rumor that the perpetrator of this Kotex caper was the nursing director of our department. The director somehow heard that I had been putting out this rumor. She pointed out to me that at her age, this was no longer possible.

One night one of the nurses brought in salmon for her dinner and heated it in the microwave. The smell soon permeated the entire floor. Jaime, the supervisor from environmental services came by and asked, "Is somebody cooking fish in the microwave?"

I responded, "We thought it was fish, but it turned out to be Nurse Vicki. Jaime started to laugh, but he had already taken a sip from his plastic water bottle. He began to choke, and we thought he might have to go to the ER. A nurse sitting nearby asked, "Hymen, are you alright?" She had mispronounced his first name. Now the entire staff was laughing. Fortunately, he recovered quickly. It would have been difficult to explain to the ER what had happened.

Chapter 56

Are My In-Laws Racist?

I met my future wife, Kathy, when I was in my first year of medical school at the age of twenty-five. Kathy was in graduate school, age twenty-four. We met at a Halloween party set up by my freshman medical class and the first-year dental hygienist class. Kathy was not a dental hygienist but came with a friend. My friends and I were anxious to attend as we had heard that the most attractive women on campus were dental hygienists.

My friends and I dressed up as transsexuals. I wore a woman's red one-piece bathing suit. My three friends wore women's dresses. My friend Dick wore a woman's pink miniskirt with a matching hat. I don't know why these items were in his closet. He wore no underwear and was not very discreet when sitting down. I have a picture of us groping each other and generally having an outrageous time. Looking at the picture, you would think we were pretty wasted, but actually, we were attending a Seventh-day Adventist party where alcohol was not served.

Kathy was at that party dressed as a pretty mouse. I thought she looked adorable. I called her two days later to ask if she would like to go out. She remembered talking to the transsexuals who had heavy makeup on but could not remember which one was me. Nevertheless, she agreed to go out. We soon fell in love, dated for a year, and decided to marry.

My wife is of mixed blood—she is part Anglo and part Saxon. Her parents didn't know what to think when she told them she was going to marry a Japanese. They asked, "Well, does he look Japanese?"

My wife told them, "No, I don't think so." Love is blind, but in-laws are not. When I met them at the airport for the first time, I could see the disappointment in their eyes.

When my in-laws saw our resolve to get married, they finally accepted our decision and welcomed me into the family as best they could. I was happy to be taken in by the clan. My mother-in-law told me, "We're not prejudiced, but on the other hand, we don't have any colored friends." I said to myself, "Hmm."

My in-laws lived in Flint, Michigan for most of their lives. Flint was then and is now made up of almost all blacks and whites. The Asian population continues to be less than 1%. I don't recall ever seeing an Asian in Flint. I think if I had seen one on the street, I would have stopped him, given him a high five, and said, "Yo, comrade."

I remember the night Kathy and her parents discussed me as though it occurred last week, even though it was decades ago. The four of us had a pleasant dinner at a restaurant called Cask 'n Cleaver. Later that evening, my wife and her parents retired to her apartment. I lived in the same small apartment complex on Cole Street in Loma Linda, California. Her apartment was only across the driveway from mine. She lived on the second floor. I lived on the first.

I stood below her stairs in the dark to see if I could eavesdrop on their conversation. I could hear Kathy's mother, Trudy, shouting at her. I have not ever heard Trudy raise her voice other than that night. I could not hear Kathy's father speak, but I assumed he agreed with Trudy.

At one point, Trudy made the point that our children would not have blue eyes. Kathy pointed out that her sister had brown eyes, and that the family adored her. That did not in any way dissuade her mother. The argument went on for two hours. Kathy now tells me that she doesn't think it went on that long. She may be right, but it seemed like a very long time.

As I stood there, my self-esteem dropped lower and lower. I continued to hear how unworthy I was to be their new son-in-law. It is something I will never forget. I was young and naïve at the time. I still had this idea that somehow life was fair. I thought if you had integrity and did your best, things would work out. I now wish I could go back in time and tell my young self, "Do not let that conversation define you. You are better than that." It is easy to accept people of all races, but it becomes something altogether different if one of "those people" tries to marry your daughter.

I would have thought that my in-laws would have considered their daughter marrying a physician to be a very positive thing. A number of people who have read this chapter have told me they would have thought that my being a physician would have so impressed my in-laws that they would have overlooked my ethnic background. Actually, my in-laws would have been more accepting if their daughter had been planning to marry a blue-collar laborer who wasn't Japanese. They have several blue-collar workers in their family who are very much loved and respected.

I don't think being a billionaire or a movie star would have made a difference to them, either. It reminds me of the threats on the life of Sammy Davis Jr. when he dated and then married a white woman. My in-laws were adults with children when Sammy Davis Jr. and the Rat Pack were popular. In 1958, interracial marriage was illegal in half of the United States. That same year, a Gallup poll showed that only 4% of Americans approved of interracial marriage.

Back then, Harry Cohn ran Columbia Pictures. He was grooming Kim Novak to replace Rita Hayworth as the next Hollywood sex goddess. When he found out the public was aware that Novak was dating Davis, he became enraged.

Davis had lost one eye in an auto accident. Cohn now threatened to have the mob remove his remaining eye if he didn't immediately marry a black woman to stifle the rumors that he and Novak were dating. Davis offered a black singer, Loray White, a lump sum of money to marry him. They married but were divorced soon after.

Davis later married a blonde Swedish actress named May Britt. Britt was immediately fired from her studio contract. Davis received criticism from blacks and whites, as well as many death threats.

In 1967, the Supreme Court ruled that it was unconstitutional to ban interracial marriage in the case of Loving vs. Virginia. I find it incredible that in my lifetime interracial marriage was illegal in a number of States.

Social mores did slowly change. The interracial romance movie, *Guess Who's Coming to Dinner*, was a success in 1967. In that movie, black actor Sidney Poitier becomes engaged to a white woman. The movie is mostly about how the parents of the couple react to this startling announcement. Incidentally, Poitier plays a nationally recognized physician, whose position does not make up for the fact that he is black. This was the first movie to show a black man kissing a white woman.

In this famous Stanley Kramer movie, Poitier's future in-laws have difficulty accepting that their daughter has fallen in love with a black man. Spencer Tracy and Katherine Hepburn play Poitier's future in-laws. Tracy is angry throughout most of the movie, partly with himself. He has been a very progressive newspaper editor for thirty years and now his best friend tells him that inside his liberal body is a bigot trying to get out. It is pointed out to him that his whole generation will have to die for society to be able to move on with less prejudice. (Tracy was in very poor health and would die two weeks after the film was completed.)

My father had been an abusive father and husband. He told me I was "good for nothing" many times. I had not thought much of it as he had said that to all our family members when he was angry. I knew he loved the rest of his family and me. However, Kathy's parents were different. These were two respected Christian, church-going members who had just met me but were confident I should not be a part of their family. I then decided, "Well, it's not me they don't like. It's nothing personal. They would love me if I were not Japanese." That didn't make me feel much better.

I have never received an apology from my in-laws for their initial non-acceptance of me. They must know that Kathy discussed their disapproval with me. My father-in-law is now deceased. In my mother-in-law's defense, she does not know I was listening in on her tirade against me. Also, I don't think she reacted any differently than most women of her generation and background.

Kathy is a strong person and doesn't let things bother her. She does what she thinks is right and immediately moves on. If only I were as strong and confident as she is.

One of my nieces told me I eventually became my in-laws' favorite son-in-law. I thought that was quite a compliment until I realized my only competition was my sister-in-law's ex-husband. According to my nieces, he left Kathy's sister for another woman and essentially abandoned his original family. Apparently, the bar is pretty low, but I still like being the favorite son-in-law.

I know my in-laws learned to love me once they got over their initial reluctance. When we have family reunions, I find that Trudy spends more time talking to me than her other relatives. We enjoy each other's company. My in-laws' love for their half-Japanese grandchildren knew no limits. It probably doesn't hurt that my daughter has green eyes and red hair. One of Kathy's siblings once noted that my in-laws never stopped talking about my children, at times to the exclusion of their other grandchildren.

Now I have a grandson named Luke. His mother is Chinese, and Luke looks Chinese. My mother-in-law adores him. It is not acceptable to admit you have a favorite child, but it may be reasonable to acknowledge one has a favorite niece or great-grandchild.

I often ask myself—were my in-laws racist to not initially accept me? It certainly felt that way at the time. I have asked myself if my reaction would have been the same as theirs if our roles had been reversed. If I were white, would I have been willing to accept a minority into my family? I say, of course, I would, and I believe I am being honest. My children are now adults and their significant others are not Japanese, and I totally accept them. However, if I were truly honest, are there some races I would welcome more than others? If my daughter came home and told me she was considering dating sites for Whites, Japanese, Filipinos, Mexicans, and Nigerians, I wish I could say it would make no difference to me, but that would not be true. I have preferences for some ethnic groups I would not admit to anyone, not even myself.

When I was growing up attending the Mountain View Japanese Seventh-day Adventist Church, I thought the Japanese were the superior race in Asia, just as there was a time when Germans thought they were the superior race in Europe. I thought the Japanese were more intelligent, more first-world, and more industrious. I put the Chinese second and the Koreans third. I put the Vietnamese, Thai, and Filipinos on the bottom as they were more third-world. I thought if you could marry a Japanese, you were at least one notch above the others, although even as a pre-teen I was circumspect enough to know that one should never say that out loud. (Comedienne Ali Wong differentiates Asians into two categories: fancy Asians and jungle Asians. She says fancy Asians host things like the Olympics and jungle Asians host things like diseases. She is able to get away with this as she is half Chinese and half Vietnamese.)

I had this high opinion of the Japanese as a child when all of my Asian friends were Japanese. When I was young, I used to tell a joke: What is the difference between a Japanese and a Chinese? Answer: A Japanese is a Chinese with a job. I was humorously showing my preference for Japanese.

I no longer think the Japanese are different from any other Asian race. I can think of several reasons for my change of opinion. The most important is that I now know "Asians of all persuasions." When I formed my original belief, all of my Asian friends were Japanese. Now, most of my Asian friends are physicians, and only a few of them are Japanese. My wife doesn't like to travel as much as I do, so I tour the world with my Chinese colleagues. My Chinese friends may not always find the best hotels, but they do get the best prices (sorry for the stereotype, but it is true).

I recently read the book: The Rape of Nanking. It turns out the Japanese were so cruel to the Chinese in Nanking during World War II that the Nazis living in Nanking tried to report the gross atrocities to Hitler in hopes he could get the Japanese to be less ruthless. Can you imagine the Nazis, the worst wartime villains ever, being appalled at Japanese war crimes? The Japanese do not have a clean record in twentieth-century history.

It occurs to me that maybe I should quit worrying about my in-laws and ask myself if I am a racist.

I ask myself if I was a white plantation owner in Georgia in the 1850s, would I have been a slave owner or an abolitionist? I wish I could say an abolitionist, but that is not likely. If I were living in Germany in the mid-1930s, would I have risked my life to oppose Hitler as he rose to power? I would hope so, and some did, but again, it is not likely.

If I were my in-laws, would I want my daughter to marry a minority and have to watch her give up some of her white privilege and acceptance in her community? It would not be my first choice.

So am I a racist? Have you ever known anyone who admitted he was a racist? I have not. Racism is subjective and can't be accurately measured. Sometimes it is obvious, and at other times it can be subtle. I would rather say that I have biases and prejudices, but am becoming more open-minded each day.

Was President Jefferson a racist? Of course he was. Jefferson did not think that blacks were equal to whites. He once said that blacks were not as highly evolved because they could not blush. Jefferson had a favorite slave, Sally Hemings. She was his deceased wife's half-sister. He knew that slavery had been outlawed in France when he took Sally, his future lover and mother of his children, to Paris when he became ambassador to France. He asked her not to run away, knowing she would be free there. Although Jefferson owned hundreds of slaves, he freed only two while he was alive, and he never did free Sally. This all came from a man who declared that "All men are created equal." He is, nonetheless, my favorite U.S. president.

Was Lincoln a racist? He was. When Lincoln ran against Douglas, he was not opposed to slavery. He was not the great abolitionist he would later become. He just wanted new states to be free and was willing to let the slave states retain slavery. Early in his career, he agreed with a plan to send freed slaves back to Africa. He only freed the slaves after the south had left the Union. At that point, he was freeing slaves that he had no jurisdiction over. He hoped some would come over to the Union side. Nevertheless, Lincoln is my second favorite president.

Maybe we should stop calling each other racist and spend more time getting rid of our own prejudices. I used to be against gay marriage. Now I realize that I was ignorant and selfish to hold that view.

Jefferson did finally free five of his slaves on his death. Lincoln did eventually become the great emancipator. Obama went from being against gay marriage to supporting it in 2012.

I am less prejudiced than my parents and my children are less prejudiced than I am. My adult children have never had a time in their lives when they did not accept gay marriage and interracial marriage. We are making progress. We've come a long way since the civil rights movement of the sixties. We have further to go, but it would be a lot more productive for me to not just look at improving others, but to improve myself. As the quote goes, I must be the change that I want to see in the world.

My late father was a San Francisco Giants fan. I remember him laughingly saying, "The only time you are allowed to root for the L.A. Dodgers is when Hiroki Kuroda is pitching." Back in the day, Italian-Americans would brag about Joe DiMaggio—as they should. My father did not think his race was superior to others, or so I thought. My sister says our father definitely thought the Japanese were superior to others. I know he was proud of his ethnic heritage and enjoyed things that reminded him of the old country, although he never really knew the old country. He only had the opportunity to visit Japan twice in his life.

When Obama ran for President, black citizens that had not voted in previous elections came out to vote for him. This is generally considered to be a positive thing. Oprah Winfrey is one of the most powerful and influential women in the world. When Obama won the Democratic nomination, Oprah said it was transformational for her and the country. It was the most powerful thing she had ever experienced. She Googled and then listened to Martin Luther King's "I have a dream" speech. She said Obama's nomination was the fulfillment of King's promise of democracy referenced in the beginning of that speech.

Oprah said she was ready to go "door to door" for Obama. When he won the Democratic nomination, she told reporters, "I cried my eyelashes off."

Oprah could have come out and endorsed Hillary Clinton instead of Obama. Many women felt betrayed when Oprah did not see the importance of making Ms. Clinton the first female President of the United States.

This has been my long-winded way of answering the question, "Did being a doctor in any way offset my in-laws' racial prejudice?" In my opinion, race is (unfortunately) of utmost importance to many people, whether they are looking at others or at themselves. It can trump both gender and profession.

Many blacks and whites voted for Obama because he was black. They felt it would be transformational for our country. A person can vote for a person just because he is black and not be considered a racist, but if one votes for a white person just because he is white, then he is a racist. Does that make sense?

When Joe Biden was running for President, he said his vice-presidential vetting committee was looking at more than a dozen women for consideration. Am I the only one who thought that Biden was discriminating? I immediately thought, "Hmm, he is saying all eligible Asian men will not be considered." If he had said, "We are looking at a dozen men for consideration," he would have been called a misogynist.

In 2022, Biden promised to nominate a black woman to become the next Supreme Court Justice. Again, why would he do that? That is the same thing as saying that if a Native American woman was qualified, or was even the most qualified person for the job, she would not be considered. In my opinion, he should have said he would consider all those who were equal to the task, and then he could have chosen Ketanji Brown Jackson.

Why was there not more outrage at Biden's exclusionary pursuit of eligible candidates? In our society, it is considered acceptable to give preferential treatment to groups who have been disadvantaged for centuries, even if it means discriminating against those who have not been so deprived. My point is, having a preference is not the same as being a racist. I hope I am not just deluding myself.

The term racist is commonly used on the internet whenever someone wants to use a pejorative term against someone they disagree with. People are quick to call others a racist or a Nazi. At its core definition, the term racist refers to someone who thinks one race is superior.

My in-laws would be racist if they thought their race was superior to others, but really they were just more comfortable being with people of their own kind. Asian parents often want their children to marry Asians for the same reason. My mother and one aunt were both bold enough to tell me that they would prefer I marry an Asian woman after Kathy and I were engaged. My late mother said to me that she did not understand why a Caucasian would marry an Asian. She did not elaborate, and I did not ask for further explanation. My mother did have several women Asian friends that married Caucasians.

It has been my observation that most white women do not prefer Asian men. That does not make them racist. On the other hand, I have found that many white men have a strong preference for Asian women. That does not make them racist against their own race.

Although I am not gay, I find that I enjoy the company of gay men. I find them to be well-groomed, articulate, gentle, self-deprecating, and tolerant of those who are different. I realize I am making many generalizations that are not always true, but I have yet to meet the exception. What I enjoy most about gay men is their irreverent sense of humor. But enjoying the company of gay men does not mean I have heterophobia. We all have our preferences.

I have decided that my in-laws were not racist, but just had preferences, as does everyone else. Besides, given enough time, we will all be in one race. I am pure Japanese, but my grandchildren are Japanese, Chinese, Hungarian, German, Irish, and a few other ethnic groups. They are mostly Cauc-Asian.

Chapter 57

Lung Removal

On the morning of my surgery, I woke up one minute before my alarm was set to go off. Somehow, my brain knew it was time to wake up. It was important that I not accidentally sleep in and miss my lung surgery. I took a moment to evaluate the day ahead. After all, I did have one more minute before I had to get up. I recalled that I slept well through the night without interruption except for that annoying nightly ritual of getting up to urinate three hours after going to sleep.

I lay there in bed for just another moment, checking to see how anxious I was. Today, a portion of my left lung would be removed due to cancer. My anxiety level was low—excellent. I had been very anxious waiting for this day to arrive. It was terrible to live each day knowing I had cancer as I awaited the day of my surgery. As each day crept closer to the surgery date, I pictured the cancer cells multiplying and spreading. Today, however, Dr. Davidson would remove my cancer—and hopefully, get it all. It would be a stressful day, especially for my wife. At least I would get to sleep most of the day under anesthesia. I was grateful this day has finally arrived.

I was fortunate my cancer was caught early. It was found as an incidental finding on an MRI scan intended to look at my heart. I was also fortunate I could get care at a world-class medical institution. UC San Francisco is the only major university I can think of that is dedicated only to health care.

The night before my surgery, I found Dr. Davidson on YouTube doing the same surgery he would be performing on me. The surgery did not look that difficult. I could do the surgery myself with enough practice. It was not that different from the laparoscopic hysterectomies I perform. As I continued to watch the surgery for thirty minutes, I started to get a stomachache. I thought this was a bit unusual, as I have watched hundreds of GYN surgical videos in the past.

The problem was that I usually visualized myself as the surgeon. I was studying each part of the surgery as though I would have to do the surgery. My wife always found it interesting when I would watch a video on a surgery I would be performing the next day. It wasn't that I didn't know how to do the surgery. I could do it with more confidence by first watching an expert who made it look simple.

In this video, I was also visualizing myself as the patient. I had to stop watching the video. I didn't need to study the surgery that intently. I was not going to be doing the surgery.

Alright, time to jump out of bed. I told myself to act cheerful so as not to make my wife anxious. I kept repeating to myself: "I know that I have cancer, but at least it was caught early, and I couldn't ask for better care." I recited a quote I had read in high school: "Courage is fear that has said its prayers."

I had had a cough for over two years and yet my chest X-rays were normal. One doctor put me on an asthma inhaler and the cough almost went away. Another doctor thought acid reflux was making me cough, but the antacid I was given did not help. It makes me think if someone has a chronic cough and their chest X-ray is normal, the next step should be a CT scan. Apparently, that makes sense in my case in retrospect, but ordering a CT scan would not have been the standard of care.

I would never have thought I would get lung cancer—I have never smoked and don't drink alcohol. I have been a vegetarian almost my entire life—mostly because I was raised a Seventh-day Adventist. I have had lactose intolerance for decades, so I am pretty much a vegan.

We arrived at UCSF, and I soon found myself in the pre-op waiting room. I was surprised to find I was still not very nervous. I had put my patients through surgery for several decades—it was now my turn to be the patient. I hoped I had been kind to all of my patients as, for some reason, I suddenly believed in karma.

When I am doing surgery, I always hold my patient's hand as she prepares to undergo anesthesia. I also make light talk to relax her. If she expresses a fear of dying from the anesthesia, I reassure her that I have never lost a patient due to anesthesia.

In the waiting room, I met the anesthesiologist. He introduced me to the fourth-year resident that would be putting in my epidural. An epidural is an anesthetic placed with a needle into the spine. I was surprised. First, I had forgotten that a trainee would be giving me anesthesia (fully supervised, of course), and second, I had assumed that I would only receive general anesthesia without an epidural. Trying not to act surprised, I asked the anesthesiologist if the epidural was for post-op pain control. He replied, "Yes, it is." He appeared very relaxed about having a trainee put in my epidural, so I took a deep breath and relaxed.

The nice thing about an epidural is that the anesthetic resides in the spine and not in the bloodstream so your mind is clear if no other medication is given. It is an anesthetic of choice for mothers about to deliver because none of the anesthetic goes to the baby and the mother can remain awake. Unfortunately, many mothers are anxious about receiving an epidural anesthetic. Through the years I have found that many women are under the false impression that if they move as the needle is placed in their spine, they will become a paraplegic. That is not true. I had no anxiety over receiving an epidural.

My wife Kathy looked as relaxed as she could. She had been keeping the conversation light as though this was all a matter of routine for us. We talked about putting my shoes in a yellow plastic bag. How long could I wear my glasses? Where would my stuff be when I woke up?

Kathy was allowed to accompany me as far as the operating rooms. She looked at me as though I was her best friend. I am. We kissed, and she left for the waiting room.

I felt at ease in the operating room. First, I would receive the epidural. I was properly positioned, told to sit, and lean forward. I placed my forehead on my arms to receive the epidural. I remember nothing after that. I don't know how I got onto the operating table. I don't know if I moved to the table under my own power or if somebody lifted me. They must have slipped something into my intravenous line.

I should have prepared my wife for how long the surgery was going to be. I had told her it would be about three hours but estimating the duration of surgery is always just a guess. I had not told her about the extra time to put in the epidural, the preliminary bronchoscopy, etc. They were also going to be using a robot in my surgery, which takes a while to set up. She told me later that after over five hours had gone by, she started to panic. She was sure something unanticipated had happened. Had there been complications? Had the cancer spread? Was there uncontrolled bleeding? Would I survive the surgery? She started to cry. My cousin Wayne called her on her cell phone. She reassured him that everything was fine, although she was almost certain that was not the case. Finally, she saw on the board that my medical record number identified me as being in the recovery room. She calmed down.

I don't remember being in the recovery room. My first recollection of being conscious was in the ICU. The fellow (a young doctor in specialty training) later told me that we had discussed my surgery in the recovery room, and he thought I was making sense until it was evident I was not.

In the ICU, I shared a room with a young woman whose illness made mine look like a common cold. A curtain separated us. At that point, I remembered I was at UCSF. Many patients at UCSF have exotic or rare life-threatening diseases and were referred for subspecialty care. By carefully eavesdropping, I learned that she had cancer and sepsis. Sepsis is an infection that has spread to the blood. I have had enough experience as a physician to understand a patient's prognosis just by listening in on the nurses. I could tell she would not survive her illness based on the conversations she was having with the male nurse who was taking care of both of us. Later, she had to have a bowel movement in a bedpan. At that point, I would have preferred a private room, but it was a minor inconvenience.

I had been asleep most of the day, so at 3 AM, I was wide awake. I was on an epidural for pain relief, so my mind was clear. I told my nurse, Guy, how I appreciated the little things he did, like covering the monitor screen with a sheet to make the room darker while I slept. He told me how rewarding it was to be part of the ICU team at such a great institution. He asked me what field of medicine I was in. When you are a doctor/patient, that information is quickly passed on to the entire team. I told him I was an OB/GYN. He told me that was his favorite rotation—that is, through labor and delivery. He would have stayed in that department, but he found that patients accepted a male OB doctor but expected the OB nurse to be female. He had decided to move on to the ICU.

I had trained at Loma Linda, which means Hill Beautiful. That medical center hoped to be a religious light to the rest of the world. The UCSF Parnassus campus is a little city on a hill. It has panoramic views of San Francisco. The Bible talks about a city on a hill that cannot be hidden. At that moment, I thought that UCSF was the greatest medical center in the world. I may have been deluding myself, but I don't think I was far off. The next day, my epidural would be removed, and I would be in pain. I knew there would be issues with narcotics, constipation, difficulty walking, catheter removal, etc. Yet, at that moment, all was calm. My roommate had fallen asleep. The unit was quiet. My room was dark except for the blinking lights on the infusion pumps.

As Guy and I looked out at the twinkling lights of the sleeping city, we shared a quiet moment of grace and satisfaction with our lives. A nurse was caring for a doctor, and for that brief moment, there was peace on earth.

Chapter 58

All Asians Look Alike

During the Covid-19 pandemic, I developed a craving for my favorite homemade Japanese dish: Japanese-style canned vegetables on steamed rice. I searched for a Japanese grocery store on the internet and found one in El Cerrito, California, thirty miles from my house.

I called the store, and a man's voice answered. I didn't know the name of the canned vegetables in Japanese, so I just asked if he carried canned, prepared vegetables in vinegar and soy sauce. He said he was well stocked with cans of Gomoku no moto. I grabbed my mask and alcohol wipes and jumped into my car. There were few cars on the highway. I arrived at the store's parking lot thirty minutes later.

Customers were greeted by an employee who only allowed a limited number of people in the store at a time. I quickly scanned the entire small market and located the prepared sushi section. Other customers soon joined me, as this was the most popular section. At first, the other customers were starting to crowd me, but then they remembered to socially distance themselves, and they respectfully stepped back. Next, I found the canned Japanese vegetables. They were neatly stacked with the picture of the product on the labels all facing the aisle.

It occurred to me that a human hand had touched each can for them all to be facing me. That is how we think during a pandemic.

I walked to the cashier to check out. I got in line behind a man whose groceries were being bagged. The cashier motioned for me to go to the end of the line. I had not seen that I had cut in line as the next customer had distanced herself six feet behind the customer checking out.

When I finally arrived at the cashier, my eyes glanced over to the next checkout line. I saw an attractive Japanese woman in her forties I recognized. Her name was Maria. She had a mask on, so I could only see her eyes. I stared at her until both of us made eye contact, then we both looked away. She did not recognize me, but of course, I also had a mask on. I thought, "Well, maybe it's not her."

As a retired obstetrician in a small community, I often bump into former patients. I once recognized a patient at our local shopping mall. I said to her, "Hi, how are you doing?" It turned out to be someone who only looked like my patient. The woman gave me a look of disapproval, said nothing, and walked away. I decided I would never make that mistake again.

I decided the woman in line was probably not my patient, Maria. We had been relatively close, and she would have recognized me if it were her. On the other hand, possibly she would only remember me if she saw me in a white doctor's coat, but instead, I was standing in a hoody with sweatpants. I had not been out of the house for two weeks and looked like a drifter.

Being seen out of context can be confusing. I played tennis every Friday night for years at a local sports club. One of my tennis partners was Gina. She knew I was a doctor, but had only ever seen me in my tennis attire. She was a nurse at Sutter Solano Medical Center working in dialysis. We never saw each other in the hospital, as we worked in different departments. One day she saw me in my surgical scrubs in the hospital hallway and said, "Hi Gary, uh… how do I know you?" I said, "You and I play tennis together on Friday nights."

I pushed my credit card into the slot. The store did not require my signature, as they did not want me to touch things unnecessarily. I was convinced at this point that the woman checking out must not be my former patient. I told myself she is Japanese, and we all have similar height, skin, and hair color. Besides, all I could see were her eyes. I would never be so rude as to say all Asians look alike–even though we do. I walked past the woman and carried my bags to my car.

After placing my bags in my trunk, I took off my mask and took my time getting back into my car. I started to wipe off each can of vegetables with my alcohol wipes. I stopped wiping, as I decided this was a waste of time. I could quarantine the cans in the trunk of my car for a few days and let any virus contamination die on its own. I decided doing that would also be ridiculous.

I was stalling. I decided I was going to give this woman one more chance to recognize me. She then walked past me towards her car, still not recognizing me. At the last possible moment, I couldn't help myself, and I yelled, "Maria!" The woman turned back and looked at me in confusion. Then she said, "Dr. Matsumura?" I was so relieved.

Maria immediately leaned in to hug me. Of course, that is a normal response when you have not seen an old friend for a long time. I immediately gave her a Japanese bow, as best I know how, and she quickly remembered not to make physical contact.

We quickly caught up with what we had been doing for the last two years. I told her that I had to retire two years earlier due to health problems. She told me how she had missed me and had found a new gynecologist but was not as happy with him. I was pleased.

As I was driving home, I recalled the first time that I had met Maria. On her first visit, she was very disappointed to find that I did not speak Japanese. Before I entered the exam room, Maria had learned from my medical assistant that I did not speak Japanese, so she insisted on having an interpreter. Although I did not think it was necessary, we provided her with one by phone. I thought Maria spoke English fairly well, albeit with a strong accent that I thought was adorable. To my surprise, the first thing Maria asked the interpreter was, "How did you get your job as an interpreter?" I was annoyed but tried not to show it.

I enjoyed listening to Maria's accent when she was my patient. I remember once she had come to see me in the office on a Jewish holiday. My two Jewish OB/GYN partners had taken the day off. Maria asked, "Why is the office so empty?" After I had explained the reason, she said, "Well, I'm glad you are holding up the fort." I found that to be so cute that I didn't correct her and tell her the idiom was "holding *down* the fort." Actually, holding up the (walls of the) fort makes more sense.

I don't know if Marie lives in that area or just traveled a long distance as I did to get Japanese groceries. I will ask her if I see her again. Hopefully, without masks, she will recognize me.

Chapter 59

Don't Let Your Babies Grow Up to Be Doctors

When I look back on my career, I admit that I am not the altruistic doctor that I had set out to be. On the plus side, the vast majority of my patients tell me that they enjoy coming to me, and I certainly enjoy taking care of them. Long-term patients eventually become more like familiar old friends. One patient temporarily moved from Washington State to California so I could deliver her last baby. She stayed with her extended family. She had been to three OB physicians. All three told her that she would need a Cesarean as her large uterine fibroid tumors blocked her birth canal. A review of her most recent ultrasound showed that her fibroids were quite large, but no more significant than in her previous pregnancies. I saw no harm in her trying to deliver vaginally again. She went on to have a successful vaginal delivery.

Despite having many satisfied patients, I have been accused by more than one of my patients of each of the following: being dismissive when they ask for bio-identical hormones, interrupting them before they were done talking, and appearing rushed.

Possibly looking back at the end of one's career, all of us have some regrets. Maybe we didn't change the world as much as we thought we would. Perhaps we didn't change it at all.

Choosing Medicine As A Career

I readily admit that I chose medicine when I was in college because it was the most respectable profession I could think of at the time. Lawyers did not then, nor do they now, get the respect that physicians receive. There is a joke that is told in regards to comparing the status of physicians and lawyers: A lawyer goes to Heaven. God gives him a house that is much nicer than the doctors' houses. The lawyer asks God, "Why do I get a house that is so much nicer than the doctors'?" God answers, "We get plenty of doctors here, but you are our first lawyer."

When considering career options in college, science was big, but technology was only a glimmer of what it was to become. I did not know what engineers did. The incredible advances of cell phones, personal computers, and the internet were yet to come.

In the 1960s, my mother took us to a doctor named Dr. Paddock in Mountain View, California. I never knew what kind of car he drove, but I pictured it being a Cadillac, which was considered a high-status car back then.

Dr. Paddock was a family doctor. Most of the doctors we knew then were primary care physicians. The disproportionately large number of higher-earning specialists would come later.

When I entered college, physicians were held in very high esteem. There was no higher calling that I could aspire to. They carried the prestige of modern-day knights. Like knights, they received a lifelong title.

Doctors were considered very noble. My childhood television shows included Dr. Kildare, Dr. Ben Casey, and Marcus Welby, MD. My favorite medical show was called Medical Center. It starred Chad Everett as Dr. Joe Gannon. Dr. Gannon was always tanned, compassionate, and decisive. He was as cool under pressure as Marshal Matt Dillon was on *Gunsmoke*.

Those doctors were always heroic. The young doctors would sometimes argue with the older ones regarding the best treatment for a patient, but I don't recall it ever being about money. I don't think in the 1960s the doctors in movies fought over money like the evil Dr. Charles Nichols pushing the dangerous drug Provasic in the Harrison Ford movie *The Fugitive*.

There was a groundbreaking medical show on TV in the 1980s called *St. Elsewhere*. It was very moving. In the 1990s, an even more compelling show came on called *E.R.* Unlike earlier medical shows, now we could see physicians with their flaws and self-doubt—a much more realistic view of physicians.

More recently, I watched a show called *Doc Martin*. I only know one other person that watches this series, but she loves it. What Doctor Martin lacks in compassion, he more than makes up for in expertise, but his personality is woefully flawed. His social skills are appalling. I find this show to be compelling because it shows that some physicians lack interpersonal skills. Of my closest physician friends, four of them have very eccentric, flawed personalities. Maybe the rest of the medical community is not like them, and I attract those types. Medical school admission requirements do not yet know how to screen for things like kindness and empathy. You ultimately end up with a class of future doctors that are exceptional at memorization and science. Hopefully, that doctor, in the future, will be able to care for a woman who has just experienced her third miscarriage. The patient may already know the medical explanation for her two previous miscarriages but is now in need of compassion.

One of my colleagues, Dr. Zaidi, loves working 90 hours per week, to the exclusion of having much of a personal life. She does not like having weekends off. When she was not on call on a given weekend, she found it depressing not to be working. Fortunately for her, she found a moonlighting job in the East Bay on weekends as an OB hospitalist. No one is recommending psychological counseling because she seems to be happier in her lifestyle than the rest of us "normal" doctors.

Two of my "flawed" physician friends are unusually condescending but otherwise excellent physicians. One is very aggressive and easily agitated, yet almost everyone loves him. Who knows what these physicians think of me? It is much easier to point out the flaws in others.

Burnout

Medscape is a website for medical providers. It says burnout has been defined as long-term, unresolvable job stress that leads to exhaustion and feeling overwhelmed, cynical, detached from the job, and lacking a sense of personal accomplishment. In their 2019 report, 44% of physicians reported feeling burned out.

The most significant contributors to burnout were bureaucratic tasks, long hours, working with electronic health records, and lack of respect. What used to take 10 minutes to chart on a patient on paper now takes 25 on a computer.

Looking back on my career, I can honestly say that I was stressed a lot of the time and was burned out at least some of the time. It never occurred to me to do anything about it. I thought it was just part of the job. It would be like volunteering for submarine duty in World War II and then complaining about the lack of showers. The obvious thing to do would have been to cut back to part-time. To me, cutting back to part-time would have been a sign of weakness. Three of my female partners have children, and except for the one with five children, they work full-time. I was the senior physician. I thought I should set an example. There is significant pressure in American corporate healthcare to see more patients. Not long ago, senior management at my place of employment decided that we healthcare providers needed to work alternative hours, that is, early in the morning or evening or on weekends. The working of alternative hours became mandatory, although they let us choose when those hours would occur.

Most physicians do not seek help for their burnout symptoms. Some say professional help would be of no benefit. They say they are not the problem. It is the system that is broken. General surgeons work more hours than most other physicians, yet they are the least likely to seek professional help. I have two general surgeon friends that take calls every other day. They have to cover three hospitals. If they are not on call, they are in the office during the day and then trying to recover from the previous night's call that evening. It would even be difficult for them to find time to seek professional help.

I complained as much as the next obstetrician when it came to things such as the fear of lawsuits, covering emergency rooms at three different hospitals simultaneously, belligerent patients, and long hours working the "in basket" of our electronic medical records. For two decades, I shared call with some other obstetricians in my town. If it was your turn for the weekend call, you worked from Friday 07:00 to Monday 07:00 for a total of 72 hours. Fortunately, there was always some downtime to rest. I often complained, but did so with a smile on my face, as no one forced us to choose this rigorous profession. We knew what we were getting into when we signed on. We chose it knowing the hours would be disruptive to our personal lives and knowing that obstetricians get sued more than almost any other specialty.

Our healthcare employer has a wellness program for physicians. Although the program is excellent, my not-for-profit healthcare corporation gave me constant grief for not being more productive — that is, not seeing enough patients. My productivity at one point dropped significantly due to my administrative duties. An administrator decided to humiliate me in front of my colleagues. I thought about making a scene and openly citing this person's personal deficiencies, but quickly decided against it. I am glad I held my tongue. That evening, I received three phone calls from coworkers who apologized on behalf of that administrator. It would have meant more to me if the offending person had apologized, but that person was young and felt she was doing her job for the organization, which she was. To me, that is the culture of corporate medicine.

You don't often hear celebrities complaining about their lack of privacy. They know that their fame affords them benefits that the rest of us can only dream of. They know they would not be able to elicit much sympathy by complaining, as it is a life they chose. Well, we physicians chose this life, and it does have many benefits. One doesn't think about those benefits when the E.R. calls you at 2:00 am.

The longer I was in medicine, the more I saw that medicine is a business and the goal of business is to make money. All the medical centers that I worked for in my career were "not for profit." Their highest priority was making a profit. Maybe this was of necessity, and I would have done the same if I were the CEO of one of those institutions, but it changed me from being a youthful idealist to a mid-life pragmatist.

Suicide

Physicians have the highest suicide rate of any profession, which is more than twice that of the general population.

The website *Medscape* estimates that there is one physician suicide per day or about 400 per year in the U.S. That is the equivalent of the number of students in a small medical school. Suicide is second only to accidents as the most common cause of death among medical students.

About 20% of medical students and residents have symptoms of depression, which is correlated with suicide, as is burnout. There is, however, a stigma associated with depression. Also, more than 60% of those with suicidal thoughts did not want to seek help as they thought it would affect their medical license. Male physicians are about twice as likely to succeed in a suicide attempt as compared to the public. Women in the general population are less likely to succeed in their suicide attempts, but that is not the case for female physicians. Women physicians are just as successful as men physicians in completing suicide. Usually, suicide is attempted by medication overdose or firearms.

The Future Of Healthcare

The Doctor's Company, a medical malpractice company, sponsored a survey called: *2018 The Future of Healthcare*. Of 3400 U.S. physicians surveyed, 7 out of 10 were unwilling to recommend healthcare as a profession. Only 26% of doctors were likely to recommend the medical profession to their children.

One Georgia physician was quoted as saying, "I am the child of two physicians. Knowing what I do now, my wife and I, both physicians, would discourage our children from pursuing medicine."

Electronic Health Records and regulations were the top causes of burnout in the survey.

Most doctors have suffered from burnout at one time or will. Most doctors complain of seeing too many patients and not having enough time to complete their work in the electronic medical records. Once we physicians entered the workforce, it was too late to turn back. We had too much debt and spent too many years training to give up on medicine and consider another career choice. Instead, we hoped to cut back at some point or retire early, although both options become challenging to accomplish.

That is not to say that some physicians don't love their work. Some do. I know several physicians whose identities are entirely tied up with being physicians. They plan to work until someone makes them stop. They say they are going to: "die with their boots on."

So what field would I have chosen instead of medicine? If I could go back in time, I would go into business. It is not as sexy or exciting as medicine. I doubt that one directly saves very many lives in business, but having run my own OB Hospitalist business for a time, I believe I would have been a more successful businessman than I was as a physician.

If I could go back and tell my younger self in college to go into business instead of medicine, I am confident that my younger self would not have taken the advice. He would have told me to "bug off." My younger self was too enthralled with the dream of becoming a physician. For a poor minority kid with acne, becoming a doctor was the American dream.

Chapter 60

When Your Smallest of Dreams Won't Come True

Like most boys who grew up in the 1960s, I dreamed of being a rock star. I would still trade places with Mick Jagger today, even if it meant looking like I had died twenty years ago. When I went to college, I started as a music major, but then a friend named Bruce gave me some advice that I took to heart. He said, "Gary, if you become a good musician, you will starve. You can become a mediocre doctor, and you'll be rich." Today, Bruce is an OB/GYN physician like myself.

Recently, I happened to catch a music video on *YouTube*. It was by Reina del Cid and her accompanist Toni Lindgren. They were doing a cover of the song "Let It Be Me" by the Everly Brothers.

Before Elvis, there was nothing (according to John Lennon). Before Frankie Valli, no one sang falsetto through a whole song. In my opinion, the greatest harmonizers of our time were not Simon and Garfunkel or the Brothers Gibb. It was the Everly Brothers.

As I was listening, I started crying—I don't know why. I don't cry at funerals and rarely cry for any reason, but here I was, tears streaming down. What brought on the tears? The rendition of the song was heartfelt, but is that enough to make one cry? Possibly it was because Reina's hair is short and auburn like my daughter's. Possibly it was because I was impressed that there were two young women, younger than my children, who loved the music of my generation enough to learn and perform it. I don't want to sound like my parents, but really, they don't make songs like that anymore.

I have a family practice physician friend, Stephano. He gets even more emotional than I do when listening to music. I'm sure we both would have preferred careers in music, but then, without exceptional talent, reality sets in. We both wanted to be rock stars, but we never verbalize that, as it sounds too cliché. Instead, we complain about our long hours working for "the man" at Sutter Health, who is actually a woman.

I sent Stephano the link to the cover song and asked him to listen. Later that day, in an email, he thanked me profusely and said we should cover the song ourselves. I responded to his email asking him if he had cried listening to the music. He admitted that he had. It was only then that I acknowledged that I had shed a few tears myself.

I told him our Green Valley Country Club was hosting a karaoke night that Friday and that we should try to sing the song in harmony. He agreed to join me.

We have played together numerous times at parties. Stephano is a "Deadhead" and I am a Neil Young fan. When we play together, he always plays acoustic guitar. I am also most comfortable with acoustic guitar, but I don't think two acoustic guitars sound great together, so I will often play bass or ukulele.

We had only tried to sing harmony together once before. We did a cover of the song, "Reflections of My Life" at a party. Our combining guitar and bass went well, but the harmonizing of our voices was just so-so. Our friend Zoe accompanied us on the violin, and that was the highlight of the song. She is not an amateur as we are. If you want to look good, bring in a pro.

I told Stephano we would do two songs at the Country Club — the first would be Simon and Garfunkel's "Sound of Silence," and the second would be "Let It Be Me." We both agreed we would practice the harmonies at home.

Stephano expressed his concern that when singing the melody, he would often become distracted and start singing the harmony with me. I told him that is why you often see professional singers in bands wearing earphones to listen to only the tracks that won't distract them. My advice to him was to learn his part well and sing loud so that my harmony would not be distracting. I assured him that if everything fell apart, and he started singing the harmony, I would simply switch to the melody. It's not like we would be performing in Carnegie Hall. Besides, the last time I had been to karaoke at the Club, the event was so poorly attended the wait staff all took a turn singing — much to the annoyance of my wife who was waiting for her Diet Coke refill.

We arrived at the karaoke venue and found the room was packed. The previous karaoke event I attended had been scheduled too early in the evening, so attendance was poor.

The first person to go up and sing was a gentleman who sang the Rolling Stone's "Wild Horses." He did a very credible job, and the crowd swooned. I made a mental note to remember to consider singing that song in the future.

The next group that went up consisted of four men in their thirties who had obviously been drinking—two of them were still holding onto their beers. They sang "Sweet Home Alabama," and as they say, "The crowd went wild." I thought about when I had watched this song on television. The band usually had a giant Confederate flag in the background, which today would be considered politically incorrect (as it was then).

Next, it was our turn. Stephano grabbed the host's microphone, and I took the second microphone from the microphone stand. My microphone had a red light signifying it was on.

For our first song, we sang "Sound of Silence." As we were singing, I noticed Stephano was singing harmony (a third lower). I had always assumed I would take on the more difficult harmony, but he assumed he would sing the lower part, just as Simon does with Garfunkel, because Stephano had a lower voice than me. Fortunately, I realized this early on, and I went into singing the melody.

In our second song, we sang "Let It Be Me" as planned. I didn't think my microphone had its volume turned up high enough, so I sang extra loud, as though I was Janis Joplin. I belted it out, and some in the crowd cheered. Our harmonies were perfect.

After our performance, I felt we had done an excellent job. I asked my wife how we had done. She said, "First of all, I don't think your microphone was on. Your songs were not peppy enough. They were soft ballads, but the crowd wants to hear something fast-paced and loud, something they can clap and dance to." She then added, "I couldn't hear you at all."

No one but your wife will give you a brutally honest opinion, but that is what I wanted. I wanted honest criticism, not patronizing accolades. That is how one improves. Nevertheless, I was devastated, and I started to choke up. "You couldn't hear me at all?" I asked. My wife shook her head.

I had memorized my harmonies perfectly. I excused myself to go to the restroom. As I walked to the restroom, I said to myself, "I know that karaoke is just for fun. Even looking foolish up there is part of the entertainment. Why am I taking this so seriously?"

As I walked back from the restroom, a fellow club member stopped me to tell me how much he enjoyed my singing. He told me he had never heard two-part harmony at a karaoke event before.

He had heard us even with my microphone on its lowest setting! My attitude immediately changed from disappointment to delight.

I learned a lot that evening. Even though my dream of becoming a musician will never come true, I realized that the smallest compliment can make one's day.

Chapter 61

Dr. Zaidi Resigns

Dr. Zaidi was tired of the more than one-hour commute each way from Fremont to her OB/GYN job in Fairfield, California. She chose to live in Fremont as her brother, parents, and friends lived there. Originally, she had applied for a job in Fremont, but things did not work out. She loved everything about her position in Fairfield except for the long commute.

One night after a meeting that ended at 9:00 pm, she decided to stay in the local area overnight rather than drive all the way home and commute back early the next morning. She asked me if she should remain overnight in a particular economy motel in Vallejo. I was familiar with the location. I said to her, "Are you kidding? Even the hookers and drug dealers won't stay there." She found a safer hotel to stay at in Vacaville.

After ten years, she decided the commute was too much. She found a job in Fremont, but after three days, decided to resign. She did not like having to share offices there. They did not offer her all the services she was used to having available to her. The people were not as friendly.

I said, "Of course, the people are not as friendly. They don't know you yet. I would live with the job for a year, and then one of the groups in town will offer you a job." She said she could not do that. Her job was her life, and she had to be happy with her job.

When Dr. Zaidi gave her resignation from her Fairfield position to take the job in Fremont, no one was willing to take her place as chairperson of the OB/GYN department she left behind. You would think someone would step up, but it can be a thankless job. Sometimes contentious issues come up between management and the doctors or between the doctors themselves. There are issues of meeting attendance, compensation, protocols, coding for billing, and mandatory alternative hours required by management. The list never ends. It is a lot to take on in addition to the heavy burden of already being a full-time OB/GYN physician.

One would think that someone would have stepped forward to take on the responsibility with over forty obstetricians in our division. Doctors, however, get tired of the bureaucracy and dealing with an administration that doesn't appear to take your concerns seriously.

Anyway, since no one was willing to take on the chair position, Dr. Zaidi was still the default chairperson—even though she had left the practice. Life goes on and decisions had to be made. She even continued to sign documents for our department while in Fremont.

In the end, Dr. Zaidi said she made the right move by coming back to Fairfield. I am glad she returned, as she is the most dedicated physician I have ever met in any specialty.

I told her in my country, we have an idiom that goes: "Better the devil you know than the devil you don't.

That means it is better to keep the job you have, even though not ideal than to take a job you know nothing about."

Dr. Zaidi then asked, "Gary, what country are you from?" I replied, "I am from the U.S. of A."

Chapter 62

Nitrous Oxide

"Ow!" I said to my dental hygienist Maria. "Do you have to be so rough? Now my gums are bleeding." Maria replied, "Well, you don't floss enough. That is why your gums are bleeding."

"Really," I replied, "you don't think that it has anything to do with that stainless steel pick in your hand that has blood dripping from it? You don't have any nitrous that I could use, do you?" Maria answered, "Actually, we do."

Maria then put a rubbery grey nosepiece on me. The first thing I noticed was a slightly sweet smell and the constant hiss of the combination of oxygen and nitrous oxide blowing across my nose. She then left the exam room to let the nitrous start working. I almost immediately noticed that I was feeling euphoric. I decided to take deep breaths through my nose and exhale quietly through my mouth to obtain the maximum effect of the nitrous. I tried to do this subtly so that no one would suspect what I was doing.

When Maria re-entered the room, I greeted her as though everything was normal. I did not want her to know how high I was. She asked me if I could feel the effect yet. I casually said, "Yes, I think it is working."

As Maria worked in my mouth, I listened to the "elevator music" being piped into the room. I noticed that I could appreciate the time between notes, something I had never noticed before. With my mouth open, I turned my eyes to look at Maria's smock. I could see the woven pattern in her clothing. Again, that was something I had never appreciated before. I then decided to look and see if she had a lot of grey hair mixed in with her black hair. I quickly looked to see if she saw me staring at her hair. She did not. She was busy looking in my mouth. Finally, I looked up at the white insulated ceiling tiles. I noticed the air holes in the tiles were of different sizes, and I tried to find a pattern.

I felt as though all was right with the world. I had come in stressed from work, but now work was a million miles away. I felt as though this was my first break from my stressful life that I had enjoyed in, well… my whole adult life. I was already looking forward to my next visit when I could get nitrous again.

When my dentist Walter entered the room, I greeted him and chose my words carefully so that I could carry on a perfectly normal conversation. I did not want him to know how high I was. We made small talk, and he asked me how my family was doing. I thought to myself, "Wow, if I had come in depressed, I would not be leaving depressed." I wondered if the feeling of well-being would last until the next day.

It occurred to me that there was tremendous potential for abuse with nitrous. I am quite substance naïve; that is, I have been a vegetarian most of my life, never smoked, and don't drink alcohol, but this experience with nitrous opened my mind to something I had not realized before. I suddenly understood why people abused opioids, etc. We all have stressful lives, not just doctors, but everyone. Everyone wants a temporary escape from the rat race or just from the general hustle and bustle of life. I could see that drugs could provide that. I could see that even though I was a prudish, law-abiding, teetotaler, even I could get addicted to drugs. I had an epiphany: I was just one bad decision away from being a drug addict.

I didn't want to go down that road, so I determined then and there that I would spend more time away from work to decrease my stress. I would enjoy the company of my family, travel, play tennis, enjoy music, and get more massages.

Near the end of the visit, Maria switched me to just oxygen to blow off the nitrous. In just a few minutes, I came back down to the real world.

I asked Maria if I had said anything unusual while under the nitrous. She said that I had asked her, "What is better than roses on the piano? Tulips on the organ." I felt terrible. I said, "Maria, I am so sorry. I should not have said that." She replied, "Don't worry about it. I thought it was funny."

I checked out with the receptionist and made my next appointment. I took the elevator to the ground floor and walked out to the parking lot. The sun was starting to set, and I felt pretty good about discovering nitrous, but there was a problem. I couldn't remember where I had parked my car. The parking lot only contained spaces for twenty-five cars, so I decided to start my search at one end of the lot and eventually find my vehicle. I found it.

I would continue to use nitrous for my teeth cleaning for the next thirty years. I have never missed a teeth-cleaning appointment, and my hygienist says my teeth are remarkably clean. I told this story to my friend Joe who is a nurse anesthetist. He was not very sympathetic to my need for pain relief. He asked me if I needed nitrous to brush my teeth.

Chapter 63

Asian Men Are Not Attractive

Have you ever noticed when you see a mixed Asian couple, it is almost always an Asian woman paired with a non-Asian male? He is often white but may be black, East Indian, etc. You rarely see an Asian male with, say, a white woman.

Asian women are considered very desirable among men (and women).

According to a Pew Research Report, Asian men are richer, more educated, healthier, and happier with their lives than all other groups of men in the U.S., including white males. These patterns would suggest that Asian men would have a considerable advantage in finding a desirable partner—but that is not the case.

Asian women are considered desirable because they are feminine and petite. Asian men, such as myself, are also somewhat feminine and petite (smaller body habitus). In other words, Asian men are often considered geeky and not very masculine. As I mentioned above and in the chapter, "Body Hair," there are many Asian/ white romances in movies, but almost always, a white man is paired with an Asian female. In the few movies where an Asian man is given the lead, I have found the stories fascinating, but that may just be because I finally get the opportunity to identify with the protagonist.

I am thinking of one particular movie I saw as a young man—*The Lover,* or *L'Amant,* in French. It came out in 1992. It was set in 1929 French colonial Indochina. (The movie was nominated for an Academy Award for Best Cinematography.) It chronicles a virginal French teen's lustful relationship with a wealthy thirty-two-year-old Chinese man. The man, just entering the workplace, is timid and lacking in self-confidence. He is committed to an arranged marriage with a Chinese woman. The French teen must soon return to Paris. Knowing their time together is short, they meet every afternoon in the seedy part of Saigon. They can hear the street sounds of the market during their lovemaking. Alas, the affair is discovered. The man asks his father if he can be with his new lover and get out of his arranged marriage. The father says he would rather see his son dead than with a white girl.

This relationship is considered illicit in 1929 because they are having sex as an unmarried couple, he is twice her age, and they are of different races. Their rendezvous are so illicit I felt as though I should hide the videotape as soon as I finished watching it. My point is that Asian men are rarely given the romantic lead with Asian women—or women of any race.

A 2005 Gallup Poll showed that only 9% of all women had dated an Asian man, whereas 28% of all men said they had dated Asian women. To be more direct about it, a study in the early 2000s of heterosexuals on *Yahoo Personals* found that among those who had a racial preference, more than 90% of non-Asian women said they would not date an Asian man. To be even more direct, or even indelicate, 40% of Asian women would not date an Asian man. (Less than 10% of Asian men who stated a preference said they would not date an Asian woman.)

Although, as a society, we have become more liberal in regard to interracial dating; we have not changed our view of the attractiveness of people based on their race/gender. White men rate Asian women more attractive and black women less attractive than average. White women rate Asian men as less attractive than average.

Black women are often thought of as being too masculine, just as Asian men can be thought of as being too feminine. I have wondered if deepening my speaking voice and giving up tennis for football would make me more attractive, but really, that would not be me at all. In addition, most of my rookie year in football would likely be spent in a hospital.

Sometimes Asian women can be stereotyped as being ultra-feminine. I have several non-Asian male friends who have told me that they only date Asian women. I find this to be particularly common among my Jewish friends, but that is just an anecdote, based on no data. My friend Dr. Jeff Katz tells me that he currently is dating four women. He adds that he only dates Asian women. I tell Jeff that he should keep that information to himself as I am not aware of any Asian female who would consider that a compliment. Jeff asked me why it would not be a compliment to an Asian woman. I told him, "Asian women might think that you have a fetish for them, that is, you like them for what they are and not who they are. I added, "They may think you think that Asian women are more feminine, more deferential, exotic, smaller, or 'tighter.'" Any of those things could be offensive to them, and people today are nothing if not easily offended. My advice: keep the preference but keep it to yourself. Be like us Asian men. If we prefer Asian women, no explanation is given.

"Jungle fever" is a pejorative term referring to those who prefer those of the Black race to the point of obsession. "Yellow fever" is a term that refers to those who are similarly attracted to Asians.

In my life, I have met women who have told me they have a strong preference for Asian men. One woman told me she likes Asian men because they are intelligent, gentle, devoted to family, and have swarthy skin. I don't think the word swarthy and Asian men had ever been used together in the same sentence before. When I think of swarthy, I think of the Marlboro man.

If I ever meet such a woman again, I would like to ask her more about what it is about Asian men she likes. I don't know if I will ever get the opportunity to ask my questions, as these women with "yellow fever" are quite rare. I think I may have already met both of them.

Chapter 64

Asian Americans Are Not Americans

The Pilgrims arrived in New England in 1620. They came as settlers to North America to escape religious persecution, but their descendants ended up oppressing the Native Americans. Following that, they persecuted the settlers that came after them.

With the exception of the Native Americans, we are all descendants of settlers of this country. Yet, for some reason, once we are settled, we discriminate against the newest group of settlers.

When I purchased my home in an exclusive area of Fairfield, California known as Green Valley, I immediately joined my neighbors in trying to keep others from building housing developments in our community. My hypocrisy gave me pause, but nevertheless, I still tried to stop urban sprawl from encroaching on "my" neighborhood.

By 1860, about 60% of the Caucasian population in the U.S. were of British origin, with most of the remainder classified as German. Whenever a new group came over, they were the latest group to be persecuted. That included the Irish, Italians, Hispanics, and Slavs.

As the end of the twentieth century approached, a new threat became apparent to the status quo. It was called the Yellow Peril. Asians were coming over to the U.S. looking for work. Although their numbers were low, a racist fear developed. The fear was that the yellow people from Asia were coming over in hoards and would threaten white supremacy. Those "hoards" included my ancestors.

That led to the 1892 Chinese Exclusion Act. It suspended the immigration of Chinese to the U.S. and declared them ineligible for naturalization.

During WWII, the Japanese-Americans were incarcerated. (The term internment would become more popular in the 1950s.)

According to author Bradford Pearson in his book, *The Eagles of Heart Mountain,* in 1944, the War Department did not want a large contingent of Japanese-American soldiers fighting in the Pacific. The War Department thought that "If a Japanese American unit were present in combat in the Pacific it would be possible for the enemy Japanese to secure American uniforms from dead soldiers and mingle with American Japanese units, thereby causing considerable confusion and increasing hazards of enemy infiltration." Of course, the next obvious question was not addressed. Why was there not the same concern for German Americans fighting in Germany or Italian Americans fighting in Italy?

If a Japanese infantryman tried to infiltrate an American Japanese unit, I can conceive of the following scenario: Bob Inouye, an American infantryman, might say to an infiltrating Japanese soldier, "Say, Ichiro, the boys and I have a few questions for you. Why is it that you are suddenly part of our unit when we have been together since boot camp and have never seen you before? Also, why is it that the American uniform you are wearing has blood-stained bullet holes in it, yet you are not wounded? And one last thing, it seems curious to us that you can't form a complete English sentence. Do you even know today's password?" Ichiro responds, "Honoruru?"

Why were civilian American citizens incarcerated in World War II just because they were of Japanese ancestry when Germans and Italians were not? My parents, grandparents, uncles, and aunts were incarcerated at Heart Mountain, Wyoming, and Topaz, Utah. The message to my parents and future generations was clear: Asians don't belong in America. They are seen as foreigners. Even those that were American citizens, could not speak Japanese, and had never been to Japan were not given a pass.

I certainly have not in my own life seen the prejudice that my parents must have seen during and after WW II. I can't recall any incident or hate crime against any of my Asian friends or relatives even going back to my furthest recollections of the 1950s and 1960s. I am so lacking in recalling any negative incidents that I wonder if I have blocked them out or just wasn't paying attention. I'm sure some of the tolerance that I experienced was because I grew up in the San Francisco Bay Area, which has always been a melting pot of many cultures, and at least from my perspective, has had a general acceptance of all races.

Nevertheless, I don't want to become too complacent and say that Asian Americans are now accepted as full-blooded Americans, as that is certainly not the case. In 2020, during the Covid-19 crisis, hate crimes against Asian Americans climbed to an all-time high, including in the Bay Area. I am a gun owner and I remember thinking that I was not above carrying my gun on my person if I felt it was necessary. I laughed to myself and thought, "Well, so much for the stereotype of the passive, quiet, deferential, Asian American who goes about his life trying not to be noticed."

I was not thinking of carrying it for my own safety. Most of the attacks on Asians have been on the vulnerable elderly (although my children would consider me to be a member of that group). I was thinking it may be necessary for me to protect the public, Asian and non-Asian.

There have been many attacks in Fairfield, California in recent years. I have an OB/GYN colleague that was attacked with a hammer in our hospital parking lot. He would not give up his wallet and fortunately only suffered a broken nose. My tennis instructor's mother was beaten outside our Safeway grocery store. A nurse from my neighborhood was robbed and killed in the Solano Mall parking lot. Her attacker targeted white women with designer purses. These are the attacks in our community I am personally aware of, but none of the victims were Asian.

Now that I am retired, I find myself in grocery stores and strip malls much more than I used to. I would not hesitate to intervene if I thought I could prevent a crime. It occurs to me that maybe with all my free time in retirement, I am becoming a vigilante. I feel as though I am becoming Caine, from the fictional 1970s show, *Kung Fu*.

In that show, the fictional Kwai Chang Caine was a Chinese Shaolin priest that came to America. He was played by David Carradine. Bruce Lee had been considered for the role, but executives at the studio worried about the commercial success of a show whose hero was Chinese. Bruce was rejected as being "too authentic." It has been said that monkeys have made more progress in landing lead roles in American films than Asian actors.

Caine was a quiet, passive man, passing through towns of the Wild West in the 1870s looking for his half-brother. He was a man of few words, yet they were words of wisdom. Caine spent a lot of time protecting the vulnerable. He didn't want to get involved and tried to settle all conflicts peaceably, but they always ended with him kicking some major cowboy butt. I enjoyed seeing whites in make-up and long black wigs playing Native Americans. Their fake Native American accents made them even more amusing. Each week, Caine would enter a new town trying to avoid conflict. When it came to race, Hollywood shows were not made in color, they were made in black and white.

Nevertheless, becoming a vigilante and protecting Asians doesn't solve the problem of racism and specifically, it does not address our failure to recognize Asians as being Americans. I say "our failure" because even I think of Asians as being foreign, having one foot still in the old world. I never understood why my grandfather didn't learn English even though he lived in California for seventy years. His wife spoke perfect English because she was born here. Apparently, he was not in a hurry to assimilate.

What is the solution?

Possibly getting rid of nationalism and seeing ourselves as citizens of the world instead of citizens of individual countries would help. Prior to World War II, Germany thought they were the greatest nation in Europe. Japan thought they were the greatest nation in Asia. I remember being an adolescent in the post-WW II years. I thought that the U.S. was the greatest nation in the world.

Since the Viet Nam War, we Americans no longer think that we will never lose a war. We no longer think that we always know what is best for the rest of the world. John Lennon believed that nationalism was not a good thing. In his song "Imagine," he sings:

Imagine there's no countries
It isn't hard to do
Nothing to kill or die for
And no religion too

Another possible solution is to stop saying Asians are good at math. I know that sounds simplistic and absurd, but these stereotypes only reinforce the idea that Asians are a distinct and peculiar people and not a part of the regular American populace.

My friend Ned Levine and I were watching the news one evening when Senator Chuck Grassley was shown complimenting a Korean American judge, Lucy Koh, who had received a promotion. He quoted his daughter-in-law, "…If I've learned anything from Korean people, it's a hard work ethic and how you can make a lot out of nothing." He followed with, "So I congratulate you and your people." Ned and I looked at each other for a second and then broke out laughing. We knew Grassley meant well with his remarks, but we also knew many would consider his comments stereotypical and thus racist. Prejudice means pre-judging. Whenever minority groups hear the term "your people," they cringe.

Ned laughed and said, "Old people are so funny when they talk about race."

I replied, "Yeah, but we are going to be old people soon."

Ned asked, "How soon?"

I replied, "I'd say 20 minutes."

Ned asked me, "Do you think it is racist to say that Asians are good at math or to say that they are hard workers?"

I answered his question with another question: "Do you remember when I told you I had read that Jews only comprise 0.2% of the population but are awarded 22% of the Nobel Prizes?

Ned answered, "Well, you meant it as a compliment and I took it as such."

I followed with, "What if I said that Jewish investment banks have done well on Wall Street, including Goldman Sachs, Lehman Brothers, and Bear Stearns? Jewish individuals also thrive in the financial sector such as Abby Joseph Cohen, Jim Cramer, Alan Greenspan, and George Soros, to name a few."

"Well," said Ned, "I'm glad you didn't mention Bernie Madoff."

I replied, "I would never mention him, Michael Milken, or Ivan Boesky."

Ned then said, "Is there any other Jewish financier that you would never mention?"

"Well, I would certainly never mention Jeffrey Epstein."

Ned laughed.

I continued, "The Hollywood film industry was founded by Eastern European Jews: Samuel Goldwyn and Louis B. Mayer of MGM, Adolph Zukor and Jesse Lasky of Paramount and the Warner Brothers."

Ned exclaimed, "Ha! I see where you are going with this. There isn't any negative judgment implied in that statement. On the other hand, whenever the stereotype of Jews running Hollywood and financial institutions is brought up, it does sound suspiciously anti-Semitic. I mean, once you bring up a specific group of people and make generalizations about them, you set them up to be discriminated against, even if the generalizations are meant to be compliments."

I then said, "I agree with you. That is why I am thinking it is better not to say 'you Asians are good at math' or 'you people can make a lot out of nothing.'"

Another possible solution is in process right now. We are becoming a more homogeneous society as we continue to intermarry. In my parent's generation, it was almost unheard of for a Japanese to marry outside of his or her race. Japanese didn't even marry Koreans or Chinese. On occasion, one would see a Caucasian serviceman married to a Japanese woman. Today, Japanese Americans will marry anyone. They will marry blacks, whites, East Indians, Hispanics, Asians, Southeast Asians, etc. The same is true of other races. That means in the future it will be difficult to have the racial prejudices that we have today. Racists will have to be very specific and say, "I hate those one-quarter Cuban, one-quarter Filipinos, but I have difficulty telling them apart from the one-quarter Chinese, one-quarter Jews."

It seems regretful that Asians will have to look like everyone else to finally be accepted. On the other hand, where you see a mixing of the races, as in Hawaii, it seems to work out for everyone.

Chapter 65

Prudence

It is October of 1970, and I am age 17. My girlfriend and I are in love, both for the first time. Her name is Prudence. She is the only person I have ever known with that name. The only other time I have even heard that name was on the Beatle's *White Album.*

We are both freshmen at La Sierra University. Although listening to rock and roll is frowned upon at our Christian college, we listen to songs that are played repeatedly on AM radio. I ask Prudence what she is listening to in her dorm room. She says she's listening to "American Woman" and another song that she doesn't know the name of. I ask her to sing a few bars. She says, "It goes: *I wanna thank you falettin me be mice elf agin.*"

The fall sky is orange from the smog inversion layer in Southern California, but we are okay with that. In addition to smog, there is the smell of excitement and possibility in the air. We feel we are on the verge of something. Men's hair is longer, women's skirts shorter. People care about women's rights, civil rights, ecology, a pointless war … and the music, the music. Woodstock just took place last year. Like the summer of love, it was something we had never experienced before and have not since. If you lived through that time, you know what I am talking about.

We're adults, and we're done living with our parents. We're finally on our own. This is our time. We don't know what the future holds, but we know it's coming around the bend.

By the spring of 1971, we had been dating for a few months. On this particular Saturday afternoon, we leave the dormitory and visit Prudence's parents in their small two-bedroom apartment in Santa Ana, California. Just outside the unit, kids are riding their Big Wheel trikes on the sidewalk. Prudence's mother remarks how annoying it is to listen to the noise that those wheels make every day.

Prudence and I both thought her parents were quite old back then, but today we are much older than they were then.

We finish lunch, and the four of us now have the rest of the afternoon free to relax. Prudence's parents decide to go to Corona del Mar beach. Prudence and I choose to stay at the apartment so we can go swimming in the complex's pool.

Prudence's mother admonishes us not to get into any trouble while they are away. She looks straight into her daughter's gray eyes and says, "I don't want you two getting into any trouble. You know what I mean."

Her parents are very cautious, as Prudence has an older sister with two small children, both born out of wedlock. The children have different fathers, and neither is "still in the picture."

Prudence and I are both embarrassed having been admonished as though we are kids. I think, "Don't they know that we can be trusted to be alone?"

We know Prudence's parents have left when we hear the screen door slam closed. We are rarely able to find ourselves alone except in my car at night. Prudence looks at me and says, "That was embarrassing."

Prudence and I had previously talked about not having intercourse until we had a place of our own, so we had never discussed contraception. We assumed that day would be a ways off as we were just starting college, and I would still have to get accepted into medical school. The possibility of unintended pregnancy was somewhat of a disincentive toward having sex. Opportunity was another. Getting caught on campus having premarital sex at our Christian college would be grounds for expulsion.

I go to the bathroom to change into my swim trunks. When I come out, Prudence is lying on her bed with only her deep purple bathrobe on. Her lights are off, so the room is dark. We start kissing.

Even though the room lights are off, there are rectangular strips of daylight shining through her louvered shutters. I am surprised at how white her thighs are. It looks as though she is wearing the white nylons that nurses wore years ago. I can feel my heart racing. Although it is a warm day, we had not been sweating up to that point. A bead of sweat forms on Prudence's freckled chest.

Things progress. She tastes salty, and I can smell a musty odor. The smell is both rank and glorious. I feel that I am smelling something forbidden. Prudence's neck and chest then flush, but not in a uniform pattern. She now has what looks like splotchy puzzle pieces of pink from her chin to her chest. Her eyes roll back. "Is this normal? Is she in a trance?" When she comes out of her daze, she is embarrassed and covers herself with her robe.

Prudence puts her hand between my legs to see if I am stimulated. There is a jump, and Prudence squeals with delight.

Soon we are lying on our backs looking up at the ceiling. Prudence asks, "Was I ..., was I alright?" I am speechless and still out of breath. I don't know how to respond. I finally say, "If you were any better, I would need an intravenous line for dehydration."

We lay there a while, and then Prudence breaks the silence. "I didn't know he could jump on his own."

"I know," I respond. "He has a mind of his own. Sometimes in the early morning, he starts thinking about you and wakes me up."

Just then, we hear the screen door slam shut. We both know what that means. Her parents are already in the apartment. Her parents changed their minds about going to the beach and came back to check on us. We would have had more time if we had heard the screen door open, but we only hear it close. Seconds count.

What happens next has to go off perfectly, as if we are trained Navy Seals. Although we never discussed it, we know exactly what to do. Prudence gets under the covers and pretends to be napping. I run to the bathroom and quietly close the door. I try to catch my breath.

A few months later, it was summer. Prudence started dating other men, but didn't tell me. She was concerned that my studies would suffer if I found out. I became suspicious and asked to meet with her so I could confront her. We met at a friend's house, and she admitted that she no longer wanted to be with me. We were sitting on a bed in the bedroom. I broke down on the spot, fell to my knees on the carpet, and started crying. This upset her, and she left immediately. I did not even date casually for the next two years.

On lonely Saturday nights, I would listen to long-play records on my stereo phonograph. I listened to this one song whose lyrics went: *Now that you found yourself losing your mind, are you here again? Finding that what you once thought was real is gone and changing.*

I fantasized that that was me, speaking to Prudence, who regretted leaving me and was begging me to take her back.

The next verse expressed my skepticism: *Coming to you at night, I see my questions. I feel my doubts. Wishing that maybe in a year or two, we could laugh and let it all out.*

My response was the chorus, *Am I lying to you when I say that I believe in you?*

This song was called, "I Believe in You" on the album *After the Gold Rush*.

I'm sure I could find Prudence again through the internet. How many people have that first name? We could reminisce, but I don't know for sure that she would want me to make contact even though decades have passed. It is still too soon. I know that I was neurotic, immature, and eccentric — still am. I don't blame her at all for wanting someone else. I'm sure she has some guilt over breaking my heart. I don't want to open an old wound that took years to heal. I just need to let her go and remember the good times.

I recall that she was a very thoughtful young woman. While dating, she once told me that when people are married, if one wants to have sex, the other should never refuse. The whole idea of that had never even occurred to me. I wondered how that would work in real life.

I know we still have feelings for each other. If she agreed to talk to me, we would both wonder what could have been. We would not be able to talk about it out of respect to our current spouses.

If I could go back and talk to my disappointed young self, I would say, "Gary, you're going to be okay. You will eventually find someone else and have a fulfilling life." My old self would say, "Well, I'm sure that is true, but tell me this. Isn't it true that there is no one else like Prudence?"

"Yes," I would have to reply. "You are correct to think that. Go ahead and stay depressed a bit longer."

My young self would hesitate and then say, "If you ever see her again, please tell her, 'I believe in you.'"

The author Lang Leav says, "…your first love isn't the first person you give your heart to – it's the first one who breaks it."

Chapter 66

A Religious Experience on the Sea of Galilee

I had always wanted to tour the Holy Land. Although I'd been to Italy so many times I have lost count, I had never seen the Holy Land. Finally, my wife and I booked an escorted tour to Israel and Jordan. It took me many years to book the trip because in the back of my mind I thought it was not safe to go there. When I thought of the Middle East, turmoil and conflict came to mind.

After we had settled into our hotel on our first night in Jerusalem, I decided to walk around and see how safe it was around our hotel. I felt safer there than I did in the U.S. I don't know if Israel has gangs or violent men, but I found it impossible to consider a Hasidic Jewish man threatening if he wore those dangling side curls instead of sideburns. To me, the curls are a male version of the pigtails that the fictional character Pippi Longstocking wore. If I saw one of these Jewish men smiling, I could not help but smile myself. I also found that most of the men I saw there had the body habitus of Asians like me, which is not very bulky, tall, or threatening.

One morning we rose early in the morning to visit the town of Magdala on the shores of the Sea of Galilee.

I could not wait to see this town as the famous Mary Magdalene was from here.

Not many years ago, Father Juan Maria Solana decided to build a guesthouse for pilgrims there. When construction began in 2009, just inches below the ground, they discovered the synagogue where Jesus taught. On further digging, they found the entire first-century city of Magdala. Coins from 5 to 63 AD have been found in the ruins.

One of the college-age volunteers gave us a short lecture about the site. She was from South America. I think her name was Andrea. She had so much joy and gratitude for being in this historical place as it was being excavated. It reminded me of myself when I was her age. Everything was right with the world. I had a purpose in God's plan. Although I no longer believe any of that, part of me hopes that Andrea does not become cynical as I have through the years.

The most impressive thing I saw there was a handwashing basin that Jesus would have used to wash his hands as he entered the synagogue. I thought that it would have been encased in a glass display, but there it was, just sitting on the ground in the open. I thought, "Wow, Jesus washed his hands in that basin, and here I am 2,000 years later handling it." I wanted to see for myself if the Bible said that Jesus taught in the synagogues of Galilee. I obtained a Bible and sure enough, in Luke 4:14-16, it says that Jesus was in Galilee and he taught on the Sabbath day. He would stand up and read.

Later that day, back at our hotel, our tour guide, Mr. Columbus, and I had a casual conversation as we looked out at the warm haze over the Sea of Galilee. Our discussion led to the story of Jesus walking on water, which he reminded me had taken place on that sea. I said, "Yeah, right."

He replied, "Wait, you are a non-believer, and yet you are on a faith-based tour?"

"Well," I said, "I am very familiar with the Bible stories, both Old and New Testament, and love being here to see where the events took place. I'm agnostic. You may find this interesting. I don't think that God intervenes in our daily lives partly because of his not intervening in the saving of Jews during the Holocaust."

I continued, "Maybe I'm like fans of Harry Potter who love to go to the Harry Potter theme parks. I once visited Dubrovnik to see where *Game of Thrones* was filmed."

"Besides," I went on, "You are Jewish, so you don't believe, right?"

Columbus replied, "I am Jewish, so yes, I am not a believer, but I also love the stories. I have this job because I enjoy it, and it pays well."

I replied with a smile, "You are Jewish."

He smiled back.

For that one day in Magdala, I was in so much awe that I almost forgot I was a non-believer.

Chapter 67

Aging Physicians

When my friend Shelly, a urologist, learned that all physicians at our hospital would have to take a test to assess their mental health after age seventy, she became angry. "That is age discrimination," she declared. "We should be judged by our performance, not by our age."

I took a different position. I said to Shelly, "It would be better for the medical profession to police itself rather than have some outside agency come in and try to set a mandatory retirement age."

Shelly then said, "That is easy for you to say. You will retire way before you turn age seventy, but I will have to take the test to show that I am still competent. Who would you rather have operate on you, an experienced urologist like me who has decades of experience or a young doctor?"

I replied, "Well, since you are asking me yourself, I feel pressured to say you. I would go on reputation, not on age. If I lived in Houston and Dr. Debakey was still practicing in his nineties and was considered the best heart surgeon, I would go to him."

"Exactly," said Shelly.

One in four practicing physicians is at least sixty-five years old. Some professions set mandatory retirement ages, such as commercial airline pilots. Most states set compulsory retirement ages for judges.

In our area, Stanford Hospital was one of the first hospitals to require an assessment of cognitive skills and a physical exam to maintain hospital privileges. It became a very divisive subject for the medical staff. When an eighty-one-year-old breast cancer doctor was asked to take a cognitive exam, he and others refused. He pointed out that some of his older colleagues had made significant advances in medicine, including finding a cure for certain types of cancer.

The counter-argument is that older physicians who have mild cognitive dysfunction often don't realize it. More senior physicians are less likely to follow evidence-based standards of care. According to BMJ *(British Medical Journal)*, patients of doctors over sixty have a higher mortality rate than those under forty, except for those with high patient volumes. Then there is no difference.

A physician at Johns Hopkins found that older doctors had fewer paid malpractice claims. He also looked at catastrophic events that should never happen, such as operating on the wrong patient or leaving an instrument in a patient after surgery. He published a study in *Surgery* that showed that surgeons age sixty and older had fewer of these claims.

Shelly was getting more agitated as she thought about the exam she would have to take in the future. She said, "Gary, I don't want to take an exam to show that

I don't have dementia. I would rely on my colleagues to watch for that. What types of questions do you think they are going to ask?"

I answered, "I think they are going to ask you to name all the vice presidents of the United States, starting with John Adams."

Shelly got a surprised look on her face. I then told her, "I'm kidding. I have no idea. Let's go ask the Deputy Chief of Staff if he knows some of the questions on the exam."

We found him, and Shelly asked, "Do you know what kind of questions they will ask on the cognitive exam for old doctors?"

Dr. Williams answered, "Yes, a psychologist will ask you, 'How are a mouse and a man similar?' The answer is that a mouse and a man are both animals. That is simple, right?"

Shelly, still angry, replied, "I would have said they both spend most of their time looking for holes."

"Whoa, whoa, whoa," I interrupted. "Shelly, let me ask the questions."

"Dr. Williams, please excuse my colleague. As you can see, Shelly is very sharp. There is no dementia here, ha-ha."

Shelly scowled.

"Do you know anything more about the exam?" I asked.

"Well, the exam takes about two hours. It starts easy and gets progressively more challenging. One of the easy questions is, 'Name four animals.'"

I thanked him, and Shelly seemed somewhat relieved that she wouldn't have to memorize our U.S. vice presidents' names.

A few days later, I saw Shelly again. She said to me, "Gary, I'm glad I bumped into you. I am still unhappy about taking the exam. To show my disapproval, I have thought of some answers that I will give when asked to name four animals. I am going to say: ass, cock, and pussy. Can you think of a fourth animal I could add?"

I responded, "How about beaver?"

Chapter 68

Inappropriate Comments at Work

I once had to counsel an OB/GYN employee of mine at a hospital in Vallejo, California. He met an attractive medical student there and made a comment that caused offense. She reported him to the hospital administration. The responsibility then fell upon me to counsel him.

He had said to her, "You are very attractive. You should use that to your every advantage in your career."

He told me that although he realized in retrospect that was inappropriate; he noted that I had made jokes and comments to him that were politically incorrect. I asked him if he was ever offended by anything I had ever said to him. He thought about it for a second and then said, "No."

I told him I knew that I voiced politically inappropriate jokes and stories in the workplace, but I would never tell one in front of someone who might take offense — which means I would never say anything like that to someone I didn't know well.

He accepted that but then asked, "What would you suggest I have said to this medical student in making conversation while we waited for a patient to deliver?"

"Well," I replied. "You could say, 'Do you happen to know what time the cafeteria closes?' You could also say, 'I hear it is going to be warmer tomorrow.' Please feel free to use either of those lines."

At work, it was time for me to get my mandatory TB skin test. The nurse who was to inject me was named Renita. She drew the tuberculin fluid into a syringe and cleaned my arm with an alcohol swab. As she prepared to inject me, she said, "Ok, Dr. Matsumura, little prick...."

At that point, I stood up and said, "Who told you? Did the urologist Dr. Levine tell you? That is a HIPAA violation!"

At this point, Renita was laughing so hard she had to take a short break.

One day, one of the family practice physicians was about to do a vaginal delivery. She was concerned that the baby was large and asked if I would be willing to stand by to assist her if the shoulders should get stuck coming out. It was to be the patient's first baby.

A nurse named Amy and I stood behind the doctor just observing the delivery. The baby was large but delivered without incident. The baby weighed almost ten pounds. The baby's sizeable head tore the mother's vagina in a line from the vagina to the anus. The delivery of the head was slow and controlled so we could actually watch as the skin parted. Because of the tear, the mother temporarily now had just one opening for both her vagina and rectum. Her doctor would stitch her back up in multiple layers, but the patient would be sore for some time. Amy, seeing the large amount of repair work that would be needed, whispered to me, "I don't know why God put the vagina so close to the anus." I replied,

"I think he did that so when women get drunk, you can carry them home like a bowling ball." Amy gave me a weak smile as if to say, "Really?"

I rushed down the stairs to attend a hospital board meeting, of which I was a member. I was late as I had just finished doing a delivery. Fortunately, the board room was just one floor below the delivery room. I quickly took my seat and tried to catch my breath quietly, but the CEO of the hospital already had a question for me. She asked, "Dr. Matsumura, please explain to the rest of the board members our new directive. It is the '10-5 rule' and will hopefully improve our patient satisfaction scores."

Fortunately, that very afternoon I had read about this rule on a poster in the nurses' lounge. The rule meant that when you are walking down the hospital's halls, if you see a visitor approaching, you make eye contact when you are ten feet away from that person. At five feet, you are supposed to say, "Can I help you?" If the visitor says, "I am looking for the lab," you don't just give directions to the lab. You take them there.

I responded to the board members, "When you see a visitor in the hall of the hospital, and you are ten feet away from them, you make eye contact. When you are five feet away, you say, 'What the hell are you looking at?'" I glanced at the C.E.O. She was frowning.

On my last day of work before my retirement, my office staff took me to lunch at a Chinese restaurant called Wah Shine. At the end of the meal, we were all given fortune cookies. My medical assistant, Sandy, asked me to read my fortune and then add the phrase "…

between the sheets." I told her, "That is a bit suggestive, and I would prefer not to say that. What if someone here reports me to Human Resources?" She then said, "Oh please, today is your last day at work, and you have said much worse things over the years. Just say it!"

"Okay," I said, "but I want everyone to know that I am only doing this under duress and this makes me uncomfortable." I then read my fortune: "Sandy likes oral sex... between the sheets." I then said, "Hey, that is kinda fun. Did I do that right?" She rolled her eyes.

Chapter 69

As I Lay on My Side Dying

My lung cancer was detected in 2017 when I was sixty-four years old. I had been planning on retiring later that same year, but decided to retire a few months early so I could start treatment.

My initial treatment was surgery. The surgery consisted of removing the lower half of my left lung. I recovered from the surgery without any complications. The pathologist said he believed all of my cancer was completely removed with the specimen. However, my cancer surgeon and my medical oncologist had both thought it would be prudent to follow up the surgery with chemotherapy just in case there had been any cancer cells left behind.

So, after recovering from my surgery, I received three chemotherapy drugs intravenously every month for six months. One of my chemo drugs was cisplatin. It gave me severe nausea. I would go to the hospital one day each month and spend most of the afternoon there receiving drugs. I would lose seven pounds after each monthly visit but gain almost all of my weight back just before my next visit. This went on for six months.

Losing seven pounds was a lot since I had started out only weighing 155 pounds. Although the weather in the

Bay Area is very mild, I was constantly cold. Kathy went to Costco and bought me some long, thin underwear. That helped a lot. She told me I was fortunate I did not have to deal with the harsh winters in her home state of Michigan.

To combat nausea, my doctor tried Zofran, Compazine, Tigan, Phenergan, dexamethasone, and other drugs. None helped. The only thing that worked was some edible chocolate marijuana blueberries an OB/GYN friend had brought me.

I always thought people were singing the praises of marijuana's ability to treat various diseases because they were looking for a medical excuse to get high. I will never think that again. For my nausea, marijuana was the only thing that helped.

Of my three chemo drugs, cisplatin had the most side effects. The good thing about cisplatin is that after receiving it, you no longer have as much fear of death. I was able to go through it once, but I think it may be better to die than to take it again.

I thought my days of taking chemotherapy were over, but my oncologist, Dr. Collier, at U.C. San Francisco, suggested I enter an experimental study. In that study, I would be given a drug called Tagrisso. This drug would just be a pill with few side effects. It could possibly further decrease the chances of my cancer returning.

Tagrisso was the drug I had wanted from the beginning instead of cisplatin, which was traditional chemotherapy. Tagrisso targets specifically my mutated cancer cells. It is known to be very effective against more advanced lung cancers. I had initially not been allowed to take it as it had never been used in patients like myself with only stage two disease. Even though theoretically, my cancer had been completely removed, cells can remain after the surgery and cause a recurrence of cancer later. In the experimental study, patients like myself received Tagrisso or a placebo to see if there were fewer recurrences in those who received the medication. The plan was for me to be in the study for three years, not knowing if I was receiving the actual medicine or just a placebo. Of course, if I had side effects, I would assume I was receiving the actual drug. I hoped to have side effects.

Unfortunately, your mind can play tricks on you. Just learning the possible side effects of a drug can give you those side effects, even if you received the inert placebo. As an OB/GYN physician, I remember preparing to start a repeat cesarean for a woman. She told me she was allergic to penicillin and the antibiotic I was giving her was a cousin to penicillin called Ancef. I reassured her that I had given it to her in her first cesarean years before, and she did not have any reaction to it. She then insisted she was already itching from the Ancef. I told her that was interesting as although her I.V. line had been placed, we had not yet injected the medication. We both laughed.

The study protocol required that I have a new chest C.T. scan as a baseline for the Tagrisso study. In the week leading up to the new C.T. scan, I had hemoptysis—coughing up blood. I had never had that before in my life. I mentioned it to Kathy. Since Kathy is a nurse, she knew this could be caused by a recurrence of the cancer.

I jokingly said, "The best thing we can do in a situation like this is to ignore it and hope it goes away." We both smiled. The coughing-up blood stopped as suddenly as it had started and never returned. It must have been caused by vigorous coughing.

I found my body sliding into the tube of a C.T. scanner in a clean, white room. I felt like a disc going into a DVD player. While lying on my back to enter the narrow machine, I noticed the room's ceiling had a poster that made it look as though there were puffy white clouds outside against a blue sky. It was a nice touch for the patient. Even though the air quality outside was poor due to fires in Northern California, the poster made it seem as though it was a clear sunny day. The things in a room you notice as a patient are totally different from the things you notice if you are a physician.

When I had been working, we had that same poster on the ceiling of our operating room for patients. As a surgeon, I remember when entering the operating room, my first concern would be for the comfort and anxiety level of the patient. Second, I would obsess about having the correct instruments in the room before the patient was put to sleep. I never paid any attention to the ceiling poster.

Whimsical thoughts entered my head as I waited for the scan to start. "How does a C.T. scanner work?" Since I am a physician, I should be able to explain how it works. I formed an answer in my head as if I were about to explain it to a medical student. "The scanner takes multiple X-rays from different angles around your body and then a computer creates cross-sectional images or slices of your body to view on a screen." I wondered, if I were a caveman, how long would it take before I could come out of the cave with a functioning C.T. scanner? The answer was never. This musing reminded me of what a colleague Dr. Goldman had once told me. She said, "Gary, do you know how a microwave oven works?" I answered "No." She said, "It is f**king magic."

The tech was friendly and self-confident as he introduced himself. He then easily threaded the I.V. needle into my vein. It was obvious he did this multiple times per day. Reassuring me that the radiation doses were safe, he then left to hide in the back of the room behind a thick plate-glass window to protect himself from the radiation.

From the safety of his bunker, he told me through the loudspeaker. "Take a deep breath and hold it until I tell you to breathe." I took a deep breath and stayed as still as possible in hopes of getting the best possible pictures of my lungs.

I had had C.T. scans before, looking for lung cancer recurrence, but they still made me nervous. I thought about the radiation exposure, and of course, one always wonders what the scan will show.

After the first scan, my body was ejected out of the tube so the tech could inject contrast media into my vein before placing me back in the tube for more images. The contrast would more clearly delineate certain parts of my body in the scan. Cancer can spread to many parts of the body, including the brain and pelvis, so the scan looks at all those areas and not just the chest. After a few seconds, I could feel a warmth in my bladder as the contrast dye flowed into my bladder's bloodstream—what a strange feeling. The feeling could be compared to the heat one immediately feels when one urinates in the ocean. Since the contrast medium goes throughout the entire body, I wondered why only the bladder felt warm.

My new research study oncologist, Dr. Andreesson, called me with the results just a few hours later. Many physicians do not like to give bad news to a patient over the phone, but I lived a long way from his office. He realized that if I had to drive to his office to discuss my results, the entire trip would be unbearable, as I would be anticipating bad news the whole way.

Dr. Andreesson greeted me, but his voice was somber, slow, and deliberate. He started with, "Your C.T. scan was abnormal. There are now multiple lesions in both lungs." My original cancer had only involved one area of my left lung. Now, it appeared that I had tumors of cancer spreading throughout both lungs. He became reticent, allowing his message to sink in. Basically, it was a death sentence. This was not the first time that he had to give bad news to a patient, but I could tell this was not easy for him.

Normally, I am prepared for bad news. In every life situation, I like to consider the worst possible outcome. That way, if the worst happens, I am somewhat prepared, and if the worst does not happen, I am relieved. I would do this whenever I received a message that the C.E.O. at Sutter Solano Medical Center wanted to see me in her office. I would always assume I was getting fired and that way I was always relieved at the end of our meeting, as that had never been the case.

This time I was completely blindsided as my scan prior to this one was completely normal and had been done just a few months earlier. The floor fell out from below me. How could my disease have progressed so fast? I had taken that terrible cisplatin for months and for no reason. I explained the news to Kathy, who had an even harder time believing what she was hearing. She always thinks optimistically. While I had dwelled on the fact that there was a 40% chance of my disease coming back, she had been thinking about the 60% odds that my disease would not return.

Within the hour of receiving the bad news, I emailed my original oncologist, Dr. Collier. My imaging studies were sent to him electronically that evening. He arranged for me to see him to discuss a biopsy of my lung lesions.

Our office visit was very grim. The Fellow in training with Dr. Collier was empathetic and respectfully quiet. Dr. Collier was surprised to see that my disease was progressing so rapidly. Kathy had many questions. I only had a few. I expressed my desire to go on the Tagrisso as soon as possible. Now that I had advanced spread of the cancer, I was a candidate for the drug that I had wanted to go on originally. I asked Dr. Collier how long I would stay on the drug. He replied, "Forever." That surprised me. I asked, "What if after ten years there has been no recurrence? One wouldn't stay on the drug beyond that point, right?" He looked at me, and I immediately knew the answer to my question. Patients in my situation don't live ten years. I said, "Never mind. I get it."

Dr. Collier told me that the tumor board had met to discuss my case. All cancer departments have a tumor board. I had sat in on many during my career. The tumor board is a multidisciplinary team that includes experts who decide the best treatment for a specific cancer patient. The tumor board has all the specialists who may be able to help. That would include radiation oncologists, medical oncologists, and surgeons.

The lung surgeon that had previously removed the cancerous portion of my left lung had commented that he could perform a very aggressive surgery in an attempt to remove the lung tumors. Dr. Collier told me that he would be willing to be very aggressive if I wanted to fight the cancer. I thought, "Wow, these people don't know when to quit. At some point, you just have to throw in the towel and say a cure is not possible. Given that, how aggressive would I want to be just to gain a few extra months of survival?" I did not want to go through surgery and chemotherapy again. I got the impression that these doctors were willing to be aggressive beyond their comfort level just because I was a doctor. I imagined them saying to themselves, "Forget the protocols. This doctor came to us with early cancer, and he is not going to die on our watch."

Kathy and I let the new information soak in for a few days, then we called our children to let them know the bad news. I was surprised to find that our children took the information well and without a lot of questions. Maybe they were just stoic. They possibly think that humans' natural history is that they die when they get to be my age. By then I was 65.

My religion had taught me that in Heaven, one lives forever, that is, we become immortal. I enjoy music but would I want to listen beyond a trillion years? What if it was mostly harp music? It could get boring and a trillion years is only a grain of sand on Infinity Beach. I enjoy tennis but maybe after a trillion years, it would be boring. I would have perfected the kick serve, drop shot, and the lob in the first thirty years. The competition would be tough because my opponents would have just as much time to perfect their swings. All of my matches would end up in a tie. I decided in high school that I could only accept immortality if there was a way to opt out after say a million years. I would want to be able to take a pill and go to sleep. I use the word sleep as a euphemism because I am sure there is no suicide allowed in Heaven.

I have a friend, Dr. Donovan. He says that when he gets to Heaven, he plans to go snow skiing, and when he gets bored, he will switch to another sport, including sports he has never tried. At some point, he will just start the cycle all over. So far, I have difficulty seeing this as a viable alternative. Since nobody knows for sure that there is a Heaven, maybe we should just cross that bridge if we ever get to it.

Living forever had always scared me more than dying and yet I was not ready to die at this time. I wanted more time on this earth.

Other than my children, I decided at that point to tell only one other person, Amy. She is a close friend and colleague. She somehow knows how to deal with bad news without getting too upset. I told her my religion had taught me that in Heaven, one would live forever. I told her that I had never wanted to live forever, but now that death was staring me in the face, I feared dying. She recommended I read a certain Tibetan book on death. She then casually asked where I thought we should go for lunch.

I read the Tibetan book. I did not find it helpful at all. I tried to yield to the concept of death as a natural part of living. I told myself I had been fine not being alive for thousands of years before I was born, so I should be fine again after my life was over. I knew death was inevitable, and getting upset about it did not help in any way. Nevertheless, I decided I was never going to be able to accept my impending death, and my non-acceptance was something I could live with.

When I told Amy the Tibetan book had not helped, she recommended that I read a book called *How to Change Your Mind* by Michael Pollan. I had previously read another of this author's books and found him to be credible and objective. The book was fascinating. I learned that by taking certain hallucinogenic drugs in a clinical setting, I might be able to get rid of my fear of dying. Drugs such as psilocybin and L.S.D. are illegal in the U. S. so I would have to travel to another country to obtain the treatment or go into a research protocol. I gave an instant sigh of relief, knowing that such a treatment was out there.

Fortunately, Tagrisso did not have the side effect of tiredness. However, I was still physically wiped out from my original course of chemotherapy. My oncologist told me the tiredness might not resolve for a year even though I was no longer on the cisplatin. I remembered that the nurse practitioner had warned me not to give in to the temptation of taking too many naps. She recommended walking instead. One day while watching television while sitting on the couch, I fell over on my side due to exhaustion. I just laid there and continued to watch T.V. from that position. I contemplated how short life was. I was born, obtained an education, practiced medicine, and was now dying. In retrospect, it seemed to have all gone very quickly.

I did not want to leave my children and my two-year-old grandson. For some reason, he was very fond of me. In a crowd, he would search me out to hold my hand. Maybe he had a suspicion I would not be there to see him grow up, and he was making the best of our time together.

There were still a lot of things I had planned to do. I wanted to help Kathy move to a smaller house. We had a lot of stairs in our house, and her knees sometimes gave her trouble. Moving would someday be a big chore. We had lived in our home for thirty-five years and accumulated a lot of stuff. We still had our children's tricycles, clothing, and high chair. I enjoyed seeing my grandson wear some of the same clothes my son used to wear. I had a 1964 Jaguar X.K.E. convertible. It would not be so easy for my wife to sell it after I was gone. She would not know how to describe it, or where to list it. She couldn't even drive it as it had the steering wheel on the right and a manual gear shift on the left. We had a five-car garage filled with so much stuff that only two cars could park in it. Our lawn had so many weeds that I had considered replacing it with artificial turf. If my health deteriorated, my wife would have to take on all of these things alone.

Each night I held my calico cat after dinner. Each night I told Peaches not to snag my clothing with her claws, and each night she did it anyway. She knew better because she would stop when I scolded her. One minute later, she would slowly start up again—hoping that I wouldn't notice. Knowing how much I loved Peaches, Kathy told me that she had a great idea. She was going to have Peaches put to sleep when I died so she could be buried with me. I was appalled. I told her in no uncertain terms that my cat was to die a natural death at the age of twenty and that it would be no more appropriate to put her to sleep than it would be to have a wife put to sleep to be buried with her husband. I told her that cats are part of the family. Kathy disagreed with me. She ran the idea by her friends. To my shock, her friends liked her idea. I told Kathy that she needed new friends.

I could not imagine life after I was gone. Should I write letters to my children that they could open on their birthdays after I left this world? That seemed morbid. Where should I have my funeral? I should have it in Mountain View, California, where I grew up if I wanted to make it convenient for my relatives to attend. I should have it in my current hometown of Fairfield if I wished my friends, colleagues, and patients to attend. Kathy said that I did not need to worry about it, as she would figure it out. I finally decided it should be in Mountain View. She smiled as she said it would definitely not be that far away and that I would have little say in the matter. Usually, I would argue, but I just smiled and dropped the subject.

Kathy told me that she did not want to live the rest of her life without me. She did not want to have to drive to family events by herself. She cried. I held her. I did not know what to say.

She told me she would cry more, but she did not want to upset me. I told her that I was also upset, but grateful for the full life I had enjoyed with her and our children. What more could one ask for than to enjoy the love of one's wife of forty years and to watch two healthy children grow successfully into adulthood? Nature only requires us to live long enough to raise our children. At least we are not like the salmon who stop eating as they swim upstream to spawn. Once they are done spawning, they die.

Still, I couldn't believe the world was going to go on without me. I was indignant, insulted. How dare the world go on without me? I knew everyone died, but somehow I had thought I would live forever. I had difficulty picturing myself as dead. Even as I imagined it, looking into the casket and seeing myself there, I wondered who was doing the looking.

Since living healthy hadn't seemed to have helped me, could I now live a less temperate life? Could I use my retirement money to eat filet mignon every night? Could I stop exercising? I decided no. Instead, I would "double down." I would increase my exercise as it helped my mental health. I would continue my vegetarian diet. I would eat organic foods—sometimes. Then I realized that eating healthy foods would also make my cancer cells thrive. Maybe if I ate an unhealthy diet, I could harm the faster-growing cancer cells. Ultimately, I decided that I would eat healthy food and let my healthy cells battle it out with the cancer cells, although I have to say that I was very disappointed with my body for not getting rid of my cancer cells in the first place.

I did not tell all my friends that I then had advanced cancer. I continued to go out to dinner with them. They told me how healthy I looked. That made me smile. I was thinking, soon my friend Dr. Levine would be told I had passed away. He would say, "That is impossible. I just had dinner with him, and he looked great." I should leave him a note that says, "Ned, thanks for being a great friend. I didn't want to worry you with the details of my illness."

Ned is one of my best friends. He has always told me to use the word Jew as a noun and not a verb. I have complied, although we have always enjoyed making fun of each other's ethnic stereotypes. We tease each other, but never maliciously. I tell him that the Jew's greatest dilemma is free pork. He tells me that all Asians look alike to him. We are such close friends that neither of us takes offense.

He has lost many of his friends to early deaths. Although he still thought I only had stage two cancer, I could tell that he was concerned. He thought about me a lot. If he was eating a bag of tasty pistachios, he would drive over to my house with the rest of the pack to share them with me. One day he was eating a pecan pie. It was the best pecan pie he had ever had. The pie came in a wooden box that said it was made in Texas. He brought over the rest of the pie for me, and I had a slice. It indeed was the best pecan pie I had ever had. When my wife came home, she asked, "How did we end up with half a pecan pie?" I told her: "Ned brought it over. His daughter received it from a movie star on the set of *Lethal Weapon*, the TV series. She gave it to Ned, who had some with his wife, then he gave it to me, and now I am offering you a piece. It is the pie that keeps on giving. It is a moveable feast."

Next, Dr. Collier ordered a whole new set of scans to see if my cancer had spread beyond the lungs. These follow-up scans included a head-to-toe P.E.T. /C.T. and a brain M.R.I.

Although I had retired and turned 65, I had not signed up for Medicare in time for it to cover my imaging studies. The UCSF finance office called me to make sure I would be able to pay for the scans myself. My two scans were going to cost me $27,000. I exclaimed, "That is highway robbery! Then I apologized for my outburst, saying, "I'm sorry. I know you are just being the messenger." As a physician, I knew how to get the charges reduced. I quietly asked for a cash discount. The billing woman lowered the charges to $5,000. I thanked her. Medical billing is so absurd. In what other field can you get a $22,000 discount simply by asking for it?

I had saved enough money for Kathy and me to live comfortably to age 95, so I figured I could afford the imaging studies since I would not need the money until age 95 after all. I was immediately reminded of a text in the Bible I had been taught throughout my childhood.

It goes: "What if a man gains the whole world but loses his own soul?"

I soon sank back into melancholia. In the book *The Grapes of Wrath*, Steinbeck wrote: "Death was a friend, and sleep was death's brother." I think Steinbeck was saying that the migrant workers in his book had such a difficult life that sleep and even death were the only escapes from their misery.

I have always enjoyed sleeping and still do, including a daily nap around 4:00 p.m. To assuage my guilt, I reminded myself that Winston Churchill used to do the same. I am sure I have some undiagnosed depression as I love to sleep and I dislike waking up. I find that falling asleep while reading a book or watching *Family Guy* on television is very relaxing, but I always wake up anxious, and unhappy that I have to get up. When I wake up, I am often in a bit of a panic, knowing that I must get my lazy self out of bed and be productive. Once I accomplish one of my chores or goals, I calm down. Waking up, one must always face the daily jostle of living.

It used to be when I awoke from a bad dream, I would be relieved. Now when I woke up from a bad dream, I found my reality was worse. I was dying in real life. I could not even watch a movie on television for more than ten minutes without the thought of my serious disease entering my thoughts.

In my last year before I retired, I was taking a nap in the doctor's sleeping room when I was called down to labor and delivery to attend to a patient. One of the nurses then told me I was always grumpy when I woke up from a nap. I told her I wished she had communicated that to me thirty years earlier. I would have then gone for a short walk after each nap before engaging them in the workplace. She said, "Don't worry about it. Even after your nap, you are still less grumpy than the other doctors that work here."

I tried to tell myself if I enjoyed sleeping so much, maybe death was something not to be feared. On the other hand, I would miss my family. Well, not really. You cannot miss anyone if you are not alive. I would just cease to be. Others would miss me, but after forty years, my friends and family would be mostly gone, and then I would be forgotten. That might seem like a depressing thought, but on the other hand, every concern I had ever had and every mistake I had ever made would be irrelevant in forty years.

Knowing my doctor would soon be giving me the results of my set of whole-body scans, I left my cell phone on my nightstand as I took my afternoon nap. Since I had worked late into the night for decades, my body had learned to fall asleep in less than two minutes. My wife and I would often talk as we were going to bed. If there was a ninety-second lull in the conversation, I would already be asleep. This day was no different. I fell asleep immediately.

My phone was set to vibrate. It went off, startling me. I had only been asleep for ten minutes. My phone said I had a text message. The message was waiting for me online at UCSF's MyChart.

I immediately logged into the UCSF website. The message read: "Hi Gary, I released the P.E.T. /C.T.

results to you. Your lung nodules are smaller, which is more consistent with infection. Please let me know if you have any questions."

I called Kathy over. I told her, "This means I am not dying. I just have an infection that will go away by itself." Kathy wept.

At first, I did not allow myself to believe the message. I told Kathy I did not want to communicate to our children the good news until I could accept what was happening. I was concerned this might be a mistake. I had already acknowledged my impending death. I was relieved, yet I wasn't prepared to accept this was my new reality.

Once I was able to accept the good news and talk about it, some of my friends asked me if I was unhappy with my doctors for not getting my diagnosis correct. Perhaps I would have been more critical if I weren't a doctor myself, but I have been confused with diagnoses in my own career. To me, that is why it is called the *practice* of medicine. We are always striving to improve.

Speaking of improvement, maybe the physician giving me the good news on my scans could have called me rather than sending me an email since the results were life-changing. The online message seemed almost flippant. I guess the message could have been worse. He could have said, "It looks like you don't have cancer after all. Have a good weekend. Go Niners!" On the other hand, I am just going to be grateful and not dwell on it. When you had a death sentence and you then get a pardon from the governor, you don't really care if the governor calls you personally. Despite his email message, he is still one of the best oncologists in Northern California.

Four months after this event, I found myself driving home from a follow-up visit with my oncologist. By then, I had totally accepted the fact that my cancer had not come back, and I was so grateful to live in a country where cancer could be treated and even cured.

As I drove my Mercedes home, it started to rain. My automatic windshield wipers came on. I thought about how the accumulation of material possessions wasn't so important to me anymore. If my car had broken down right then, and I had to walk home, normally I would have found that to be upsetting. However, in light of recent events, I would have been fine walking home with the rain on my face. As I drove home, there was still light in the sky, and rather than anticipating the future, I just enjoyed the moment.

I sent a draft of this chapter to my Nurse Anesthetist friend. He is also a former Marine. We had worked together for two decades in labor and delivery until he retired. As he read my story, he became upset and started crying. Even when he finished the story and saw that I was not dying, he could not stop crying. He called me on the phone to express his displeasure with me for upsetting him, but I could tell he was relieved to know that I would survive my cancer. He asked me if I was cured. I told him, "I think I am cured, but cancers have been known to recur even twenty years after they were treated. Nevertheless, I'm going to say that I'm cured."

Chapter 70

Nearly a Near-Death Experience

Near-Death Experience (NDE) as described in the media would generally not refer to my experience of thinking I was going to die soon and then receiving a reprieve. NDE more often refers to someone who had an acute episode in which they may have actually died but then were revived such as after a heart attack or drowning. Those that experience an NDE often describe a feeling of floating above their body, meeting spiritual beings such as angels, entering a tunnel, and seeing a bright light. They often have a sense of peace and of being loved unconditionally. Some encounter deceased loved ones. They are ultimately called from that realm and back into their own body. These people often feel more compassionate towards others after the event. They are more altruistic and less materialistic.

Everyone does not come out of this experience in a positive way. Less commonly, one can have post-traumatic stress disorder such as when someone is almost killed in combat.

Those that survive a cardiac arrest are sometimes more self-assured, socially aware, and religious than before the event. They have a reduced fear of death and have less concern for material gain or status. Well, that would all make sense. If you can see that life is not just about you, but your place in the greater universe, and that death is not something to be feared, but a pleasant experience, then your outlook would be changed for the better. Life becomes more meaningful and fulfilling.

These people often say they are no longer afraid of dying. But that doesn't mean they are more prone to commit suicide. On the contrary, they are much less suicidal than those who have not had an NDE. When asked why that is, they say that when you lose your fear of death, you also lose your fear of life. You are no longer afraid of losing everything. You are willing to take chances and live life to the fullest.

My simple view of someone who had an NDE would be someone whose heart stopped and was unconscious but somehow came back to life.

I would consider my experience to be more of a close brush with death or a near-death situation. I didn't actually experience death and come back, so I would assume that my experience would not be as profound. Nevertheless, I feel as though I have changed in some ways.

I have been forced to confront what is and is not important in life. One of the consequences of this is that I am starting to distribute some of my wealth now rather than waiting for it to be dispersed at my death. Why not start helping people now rather than later? By the time I die, maybe those recipients won't need help.

Just as those who have had an NDE felt less fear of death, I also am more at peace with the concept, even though I don't feel more religious. Having gone through a dress rehearsal of preparing for death, I feel I will be more prepared for it when my time comes. In other words, having to deal with a life-threatening experience has made me better prepared for the next one.

I thought that having looked death in the face and then being given a second chance to live a healthy life again, I would be less materialistic. I told myself that now I would not care if I was driving my new Tesla Y or if I were driving my old 1972 Plymouth Duster. It would make no difference to me in the total picture of things. But then I thought I would really miss my heated seats. Also, having a blind-spot warning system to help you change lanes isn't really a luxury. For me, it is a necessity. I can ask my radio to play any song and it does.

I still enjoy trading stocks just as much now as when I entered the workforce in 1982. I enjoy watching my stocks go up and feel angst when they go down, although it really makes no difference to me, as I will remain comfortably retired no matter what the stock market does. So maybe I am just as materialistic as I was before, but I have changed in other ways.

I feel as though I am living now more in the present and not always worrying about the future. When I place my cat Peaches on my lap, I tell her how much I appreciate our friendship. I think less about her growing old and her future. Unlike all my previous cats, Peaches could outlive me.

Having thought a lot about death recently, I now realize that death does not have to be unpleasant. Doctors are often able to make us comfortable with medications at the end of life. Whether the experience of death as described by those who have experienced an NDE is real or imagined, either way it is still pleasant. It is about being surrounded by loved ones. It is escorted and guided. I used to think death was going to be terrible. I feared I would be in a hospital, possibly on a respirator. Actually, it may be beautiful, even ecstatic. The last words from Steve Jobs were: "Oh wow. Oh wow. Oh wow."

We are never closer to life than when we brush up against the possibility of death. Getting a second chance at living is like hitting the reset button. You get to start a new life. Laura Ingalls Wilder published her first *Little House* book at age 65. I feel young at heart. I hope to start a new career as a writer.